Motor Neurone Disease

(Amyotrophic Lateral Sclerosis)

Sue Beresford

Head Occupational Therapist
Northampton General Hospital
Northampton
UK

Consultant editor: Jo Campling

CHAPMAN & HALL

London · Glasgow · Weinheim · New York · Tokyo · Melbourne · Madras

Published by Chapman & Hall, 2–6 Boundary Row, London SE1 8HN, UK

Chapman & Hall, 2–6 Boundary Row, London SE1 8HN, UK

Blackie Academic & Professional, Wester Cleddens Road, Bishopbriggs, Glasgow G64 2NZ, UK

Chapman & Hall GmbH, Pappelallee 3, 69469 Weinheim, Germany

Chapman & Hall USA, 115 Fifth Avenue, New York NY 10003, USA

Chapman & Hall Japan, ITP-Japan, Kyowa Building, 3F, 2-2-1 Hirakawacho, Chiyoda-ku, Tokyo 102, Japan

Chapman & Hall Australia, 102 Dodds Street, South Melbourne, Victoria 3205, Australia

Chapman & Hall India, R. Seshadri, 32 Second Main Road, CIT East, Madras 600 035, India

Distributed in the USA and Canada by Singular Publishing Group Inc., 4284 41st Street, San Diego, California 92105

First edition 1995

© 1995 Sue Beresford

Phototypeset in 10/12 pt Times by Intype, London

Printed in England by Clays Ltd, St Ives plc

ISBN 0 412 55640 5   1 56593 318 4 (USA)

A catalogue record for this book is available from the British Library

Library of Congress Catalog Card Number: 95–69063

∞ Printed on permanent acid-free text paper, manufactured in accordance with ANSI/NISO Z39.48–1992 and ANSI/NISO Z39.48–1984 (Permanence of Paper).

Peace comes to them that wait

Inside outside everything is strange
Can't reach inside my pocket to get my change
Never realised what I would become
Never thought I would see my son
This damn disease it keeps getting worse
All I can look forward to is a trip in a hearse
I think of the years all gone past falling away
from me
I think of James and what he might be
If I can leave one thing here on this earth
It will have to be my very last breath
Some say life is what you make it and I had my
fun
I believe there is no Hell only life above the Sun
If I could have one last request it would be from
God
To look after the ones I have loved and not hate
me for being a sod

Alex Q. Buchanan (1994)

Contents

Foreword

Motor neurone disease (MND) was described by the French physician Charcot 120 years before this book was written. But for most of that time it was regarded by scientists as a rare disease of little interest, and by the medical profession with frank defeatism. Standard reference works dismissed the disease in a few lines; as being of unknown aetiology, with no available treatment and a dismal prognosis. This assessment was devastatingly accurate; the lot of most people diagnosed with MND was indeed one of helpless misery for them and for their carers. There were a few exceptions in the last generation: Kurland and Norris in the USA, Saunders and Clifford Rose in the UK; these and a handful of others had an altogether more robust view of the potential of an active response to MND.

Many unspeakable diseases known to medical science are still beyond the reach of fundamental treatment. MND must take its place in the first rank. Paralysing the body but generally leaving the intellect untouched, rapidly progressive with a life expectancy of a few months to a few years from definite diagnosis, with new and cruel disabilities following the loss of each muscle function. The disease rapidly saps the physical resources of patients, and of their immediate carers. It drains their emotional and financial resources too, and can quickly exhaust their wider social network, literally as well as figuratively. It heaps one indignity upon another, reducing the healthy adult to infant inability to clean themselves or control secretions. Learning to cope with a disease about which most people never expect to have to learn is one thing. But MND simultaneously forces patient and carers to attempt to learn the labyrinthine complexities of the equally unfamiliar health and social care systems.

All this began to change in the 1970s with the simultaneous emergence in many countries of voluntary associations, driven by patients and carers who refused to be defeated by this many-headed monster. By the time this book was written, there were over 400 major associations in more than 30 countries, of which the largest was the Motor Neurone Disease

Association of the UK, followed by the ALS Association in the USA. The associations saw it as their role to provide information, to give practical help and support to as many patients and families as possible, and to fund research. They saw as their natural partners the physicians and therapists whose work routinely brought them into contact with people with MND. Novel collaborations sprang up in which multidisciplinary teams included as equals the neurologists, therapists, nurses, social workers, volunteers and carers – and the patients themselves. For this is a disease in which the patient above all is the expert. Only he/she can say how much loss of dignity is worth the retention of how much autonomy, only he/she can say when the point of diminishing returns is reached between discomfort and dependence.

By the beginning of the 1990s the first causal factors in MND had been identified through advances in molecular genetics. Simultaneously the biochemistry of MND has been unravelled far enough for the first clinical trials of possible drug treatments to begin to yield hopeful results. Informed opinion suggests that MND will be shown to be a complex, multifactorial disease, and that no single cause will be found that would readily respond to treatment. Postponing the onset of certain disabilities or delaying death through major advances in themselves would not end the suffering brought by MND.

Substantial improvements in the quality of life would instead result from enlightened management of the disease, and care of the patient and family. The capricious nature of MND exerts its own disciplines; nevertheless, appropriate and timely symptom control and palliative measures; humane and ethical introduction of life support technology; appropriate emotional and psychological support; the application of evolving thera- peutic practices; and above all, patient-centred care – all these, borrowed from many other disciplines and diseases, and applied in a planned and proactive way, can help to ensure that the life that remains is at least tolerable, but at its best can be creative and fulfilling.

Peter Cardy,
Director, Motor Neurone Disease Association UK
Secretary General, International Alliance of ALS/MND Associations

Acknowledgements

I would like to thank the following people for their help and support during the preparation of this book:

The families with whom I have worked for allowing me to use their stories; special thanks to Alex Buchanan for permission to publish his poem. Drs Peter Kaye and John Smith, Consultants in Palliative Medicine, Jenny Hill, Senior Day Unit Nurse, and Barbara Malcolmson, Senior Physiotherapist, Cynthia Spencer House, Northampton; Peter Cardy, Director, Tricia Holmes, Director of Operations, Jane Skelton, Regional Care Advisor, and the Northants Branch, MNDA, for their help and contributions to this work. My family, John, Stuart and Mark for their patience and finally to Jo Campling and the staff of Chapman & Hall for their encouragement and direction.

Author's note

I have always felt uncomfortable referring to people as patients but, for ease of writing, it is less clumsy than some other phraseology. For this reason also, I refer to the patient as 'he' and carers and healthcare professionals as 'she' throughout the text.

PART ONE

Motor Neurone Disease – a Description

Motor neurone disease

> Whatever else you do, don't get motor neurone disease,
> it's bloody ghastly.
>
> (*David Niven*)

INTRODUCTION

David Niven died in 1983, after suffering for some time from motor neurone disease (MND). The television news at the time reported that he had died from a muscle wasting illness, but it was not named and few people had heard of MND. In 1993, a family coping with the effects of MND was the focus of a three-part television drama series and many more people are now aware of the illness. Motor neurone disease has been medically recognized for 120 years but it is only in the last ten years that awareness of the illness has increased and the need for improved patient care has been addressed.

Research is being carried out into the possible cause of MND and gradually more is being understood about the illness, its effects and the needs of those who suffer from it. Since this book was conceived, scientists have confirmed a genetic link in the familial form of MND. A cure still lies some way ahead but gradually the hope that one will be found becomes clearer.

Motor neurone disease is a progressive degenerative disease affecting the motor neurones in the corticospinal pathways, as well as those in the motor nuclei of the brainstem and the anterior horn cells of the spinal cord (Figure 1.1). The autonomic nervous system and the sensory nerves are unaffected. Intellect and memory remain intact throughout.

In some parts of the world, particularly the USA, the condition is known as amyotrophic lateral sclerosis (ALS). In the UK, the term 'motor neurone disease' is used to describe the degenerative condition of which ALS is a specific type. This can give rise to some confusion.

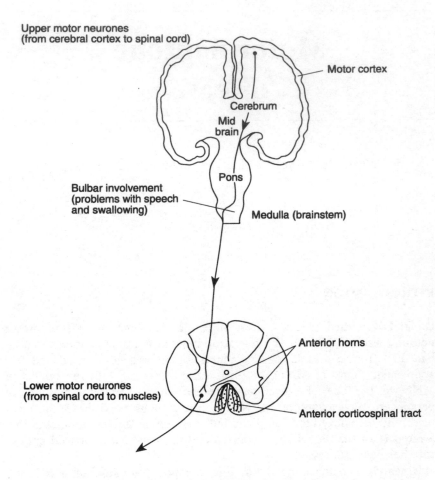

Figure 1.1 Brain and cross-section of spinal cord, illustrating areas affected by motor neurone disease.

DESCRIPTION OF MOTOR NEURONE DISEASE

There are thought to be three main types of the disease. They rarely occur exclusively, and whilst a person may present initially with one type, he may later develop a combination of two or all three types of the disease. The symptoms at the onset are often asymmetrical. Differentiation at the time of diagnosis may give an indication of prognosis.

Amyotrophic lateral sclerosis (ALS)

This is the most common form of MND and affects about 80% of people with the disease. ALS affects the upper motor neurones predominantly, although lower motor neurones may also be affected. If the latter is the case, fasciculations (muscle twitching under the skin) will be noticed.

The most common presenting symptom of this type of MND is weakness of the small muscles of the hand or an asymmetrical foot drop. Regular night cramps, particularly in the calf muscles, may also be experienced. As the disease progresses, spasticity and muscle weakness can impair walking and spasms may also be particularly troublesome at night. Where the upper motor neurones are affected, reflexes can become more brisk. Prognosis is thought to be between three and five years from diagnosis.

Progressive muscular atrophy (PMA)

In this type of the disease, the lower motor neurones are affected most severely. The initial signs are often wasting in the small muscles of the hands and feet. Fasciculations are particularly associated with the destruction of the lower motor neurones. Weakness usually begins in the extremities and works its way towards the body but, occasionally, weakness may begin in the shoulder joints.

This type of the disease affects about 8% of people with the illness and the prognosis is thought to be better than that for the other types of the disease, with many people living longer than five years and some surviving for more than 20 years. The prognosis may, however, be reduced if bulbar signs are present.

Progressive bulbar palsy (PBP)

PBP affects the tongue, the muscles of the palate, pharynx and larynx. The muscles of the face may also be involved, as often are the muscles of the shoulder girdle and arms. Fasciculations and wasting of the tongue may be present. It is quite common for the speech to be completely lost and swallowing to be badly affected whilst the person is still able to walk around.

Progressive bulbar palsy carries the worst prognosis, between six months and three years from diagnosis. The severity of muscle weakness in the areas vital to life, such as breathing and swallowing, is usually the determining factor.

Familial MND

In general, MND is not an inherited condition but in a few cases (between 5 and 10%) a familial link can be traced. The link can usually be traced back through several generations of the family, where relatives have often died from a form of progressive paralysing illness, undiagnosed at the time, but later understood to be MND.

MND does not usually affect the intellect but, in some cases of familial MND, dementia has been observed. Mulder and Kurland (1987) also relate that cerebellar disease, Huntington's chorea and occasionally Parkinsonism have been known to occur with familial MND.

It is thought that the age of onset of the familial form of MND may be earlier than that of the sporadic form but otherwise, the clinical picture is the same. Where the familial form occurs, genetic counselling is usually offered to other members of the family where appropriate.

PROGRESSION OF MOTOR NEURONE DISEASE

ALS and PMA

The speed of progression and areas of spread of the disease are unpredictable in both of these types of MND. Muscle weakness may be unilateral at the onset of the illness but invariably spreads bilaterally affecting muscles in the limbs, the trunk and the neck. Often some muscle power remains in a muscle group as the illness progresses to another part of the body, but may be lost later in the illness.

Speech is usually affected to some degree during the progression of the illness (Saunders, Walsh and Smith, 1981). This can vary from loss of volume as a result of breathing difficulties to total lack of speech caused by additional bulbar signs.

There are no remissions as such but the speed of progression of the disease may appear to vary, with a period of deterioration followed by a period of comparative stability in the condition, lasting for some weeks or months. It is known that muscles can still be activated by relatively few motor neurones and sudden deterioration may be the result of destruction of a few neurones, vital to keeping specific muscles working.

PBP

The progression of PBP differs from the other two types of MND primarily because of the muscle groups that are affected. Slurring of speech, difficulty controlling saliva and swallowing are the most usual initial symptoms. This is often followed by weakness and wasting in the muscles of the shoulder girdle, chest, diaphragm and upper arms and then weakness and wasting in the forearm and hand.

If the muscles associated with breathing are severely affected, poor basal expansion can lead to serious chest infections, pneumonia or respiratory failure, which can prove fatal. In a few cases, people initially diagnosed as having predominantly bulbar signs can go on to develop signs of the other types of MND as well.

INCIDENCE

The annual incidence of MND is approximately 1:50 000 of the population, which is similar to the number of people suffering from multiple sclerosis (MS). The prognosis of MND is worse than that of MS so the prevalence of MND is thought to be 8–10 sufferers per 100000 of the population against 50 in 100000 of the population who suffer from MS.

The average age of onset is thought to be between 50 and 70 years of age. The disease rarely affects people under 40 years or older than 80 years (Newrick and Langton-Hewer, 1984; O'Brien, Kelly and Saunders, 1992) and males are affected slightly more frequently than females in a ratio of 1.6:1 (Mulder and Kurland, 1987). It is generally agreed that in recent years, the average age of onset may have reduced, as more people in the 20–40 year age group are now affected than was documented in earlier years.

CLINICAL FEATURES

MND can affect any of the muscles under voluntary control leading to weakness and wasting of the muscles and general fatigue of the patient. Initially, weakness can be out of proportion to the loss of movement and, at rest, many patients relate that they feel well in themselves until they try to move and find they are unable to do so.

In general, the sensory nervous system is not involved; however, Mulder and Kurland (1987) found that 'specific testing reveals that in about 20% of patients with MND, sensory findings can be demonstrated'. It is not unusual for patients to relate that they have altered sensation in certain areas of the body; however, some people find it difficult to differentiate sensory involvement from motor impairment.

Uncontrollable laughter and tears may result if upper motor neurones are involved, particularly in the bulbar region. This mechanical response can cause alarm to patients if not explained, since the patient may fear psychological or psychiatric illness to be the cause.

Erratic temperature control, although not documented as a usual problem with this illness, is often present. Many patients have related a propensity for feeling excessively hot, excessively cold or a swing between the two. This can usually only be controlled by controlling the temperature of the environment in which the patient lives.

Sight, hearing, touch and taste remain intact. The nerves linked to eyeball movement are rarely affected and can be used as a basis for communication if speech is lost. The eyelids may blink less frequently causing the eyes to feel gritty.

Bladder and bowel control are not affected by MND despite the level of muscle weakness experienced, since sphincter muscles are not affected by the disease. Careful attention to bowel management can prevent constipation which may occur as the patient becomes less mobile, particularly if abdominal muscles weaken and the diet contains less fibre as a result of eating difficulties.

MND does not alter a person's intellect or memory, but living with the psychological problems that it involves can place severe pressure on the person's personality and coping mechanisms. This can result in the person behaving in ways that may be out of character, and can lead family members to conclude that the illness affects mental function. In a small number of people (usually those suffering from the familial type of MND), dementia or mental impairment may be present.

Sexual function is rarely affected although it may be lost in the later stages of the illness where muscle weakness is pronounced. Creativity of thought may be necessary to maintain intimacy as muscles become weaker.

DIAGNOSIS

There are no specific tests that can be administered to determine conclusively a diagnosis of MND. Diagnosis is invariably clinical, there being certain signs which will suggest a diagnosis of MND to the physician. Combined upper and lower motor neurone degeneration without sensory loss, fasciculations (twitching) of the muscles, unexplainable speech and swallowing difficulties or marked wasting of the muscles may be present.

Investigations may be carried out to support or refute the clinical findings. Blood tests are usually found to be normal but may, in a few cases, show raised blood creatinine kinase levels. Examination of cerebrospinal fluid may show raised protein level but is often normal.

Electrophysiological investigations can, however, be more useful. Electromyography records the electrical changes found in muscles at rest and during voluntary movement. Denervation and fasciculation potentials are characteristic findings in a positive diagnosis of motor neurone disease. If the picture is still obscure, further investigations may be necessary to exclude other neurological conditions.

CAUSES

At present, the cause of MND is not known. Research is being carried out at various centres in Britain and other parts of the world in an attempt to find out why some people develop the disease and others do not. Research is focused on:

1. discovering the cause of the illness – whether genetic or environmental;
2. the possibility that motor neurones may be encouraged to regrow;
3. attempts to arrest the progression of motor neurone deterioration;
4. improvement of patient care by development of an improved range of equipment to aid daily living.

TREATMENT

At present there is no known cure for MND. However, control of unpleasant symptoms and effective management of care for people with the disease are vital. If carried out efficiently, symptom control can improve the quality of life experienced by the person with the disease and their family and empathetic care management enables patients to have more control over their lives than would otherwise be possible in this situation.

Symptom control is a medical speciality and most people with MND experience some unpleasant symptoms, however mild, through the progression of their illness. In some areas of the country symptom control is carried out by a neurological consultant; in others it is the province of the consultant in palliative medicine.

General practitioners usually have little experience of motor neurone disease and are unsure of many of the treatments available to reduce unpleasant symptoms. The patient and family gain considerable reassurance from the knowledge that they have access to a senior medical practitioner who knows about the illness should the need arise, and can advise on symptom control.

CONCLUSION

Motor neurone disease is a progressive neuromuscular illness for which there is, as yet, no cure. People can be led to believe that since a cure has not been found, no treatment can be offered. Most unpleasant symptoms can be improved by good palliative care, and empathetic support can help the patient and family to cope with the physical and emotional effects of this disease.

REFERENCES

Mulder, D. W. and Kurland, L. T. (1987) Motor neurone disease: epidemiological studies. *Ad. Exp. Med. Biol.*, **209**, 325–32.

Newrick, P. G. and Langton-Hewer, R. (1984) Motor neurone disease: can we do better? A study of 42 patients. *B.M.J.*, **289**, 539–42.

O'Brien, T., Kelly, M. and Saunders, C. (1992) Motor neurone disease: a hospice perspective. *B.M.J.*, **304**, 471–3.

Saunders, C., Walsh, T. D. and Smith, M. (1981) Chapter 6 in *Hospice – The Living Idea*, (eds D. H. Summers, C. Saunders and N. Teller), Edward Arnold, London, p. 131.

FURTHER READING

Bannister, Roger (1985) *Brain Clinical Neurology* (revised edn), Oxford University Press, London.

Cochrane, G. M. (ed.) (1987) *The Management of Motor Neurone Disease*, Churchill Livingstone, Edinburgh.

Cochrane, G. M. (1989) Motor neurone disease. *British Journal of Hospital Medicine*, **41**, March.

MNDA Annual Report 1992–93, Motor Neurone Disease Association, Northampton.

Schwartz, M. S. and Swash, M. (1992) *Motor Neurone Disease*, in *Neurology*, Churchill Livingstone, Edinburgh.

PART TWO

The Multidisciplinary Approach

There is too a deeply contemplative aspect to the work for it demands not just that we do things for people but that we be with them. It is a ministry of presence, a being alongside the suffering, impotent as they are impotent, mute as they are mute, sharing their darkness.

(Cassidy, 1988).

People who work in hospices or palliative care units do so because they are called to the work. Many try for a while but then decide it is not for them; others continue for some years to work alongside these people as part of the team. Palliative care does not appeal to everyone but occasionally when working as part of a community team, any health professional may be required to work with a client who is terminally ill.

People with MND may live for some years with a slowly declining capability but, in the UK where the use of mechanical ventilation is rare, their death usually results from the effects of the illness. This requires that through the course of the disease, attention is paid to issues relating to living with terminal illness.

This section looks at the work of the multidisciplinary team which may be based in the community, a hospital, hospice or residential home It aims to explain why a multidisciplinary approach is necessary and suggests a theoretical base from which to begin.

Health and social services are in a time of rapid and radical change. They are now required to act from autonomous units within the whole, purchase and provide care from different areas of the service, and each unit must be accountable for its own budget. Where once health and social care were offered to all, regardless of their ability to contribute financially, we are now entering an era where people are expected more and more frequently to contribute towards the cost of their care.

Accurate assessment of a person's needs is vital to ensure that they receive good quality, cost-effective care. Continual reassessment is necessary with this patient group to identify changes in circumstance and ensure that the correct level of care is maintained. In a world where more emphasis is placed upon cost efficiency, this aspect of community care is becoming increasingly more important.

Caring for people with MND and their families requires an holistic approach to assessment and provision of services. Ways in which this can be achieved by the multidisciplinary team are addressed here.

The multidisciplinary team

You give but little when you give of your possessions.
It is when you give of yourself that you truly.give.
(Gibran, 1991).

INTRODUCTION

MND affects many of the functions in the body. In order to provide effective care and treatment, an holistic approach has been found to be most appropriate. A team of people working together can address different needs at different stages of the illness and provide the best overall care.

For the health professional, working with a patient and family who are coping with MND can be stressful, whether they are cared for in the community or in a residential setting. The illness is unpredictable, unrelenting and can progress over many months or years. Functioning within a team can provide support for team members when pressure mounts.

TEAMWORK

The *Oxford Modern English Dictionary* defines teamwork as 'the combined action of a team, group, etc. especially when effective and efficient'. In order for the team to achieve effectiveness and efficiency, it must have a common goal – in effect it aims to solve a common problem. The team functions best under the guidance of a sensitive leader or team manager.

Working as a team member in this area of care involves helping people to face life-threatening situations. This will necessitate that the health professional give consideration to thoughts and feelings about her own morality. Feelings associated with this area of concern may be frightening to some people, who may be reluctant to address the issues to which they relate. Failure to do this usually causes problems for the health professional at a later date, and time should be allowed to work through and explore these issues as they arise.

Particular difficulties associated with the progression of the illness may be experienced. The disease process is unpredictable so input may be required over many months or years. This will require the therapeutic relationship to last throughout this period of time. However positive the approach of the health professional, there will be times when watching the slow deterioration of the patient can be painful and distressing.

Many of the bodily functions are affected by the illness and, as a result, the team of people who may be needed to advise and care for the patient and carer may be large. It may also require the input of a number of different teams, working in co-ordination. Wherever the team is functioning, it will centre around the patient and carer and the ultimate aim will be to assess and provide for their care needs.

DIFFERENT TEAMS THAT MAY BE INVOLVED

Community

The community team may include the general practitioner, district nurse, community occupational therapist, community physiotherapist, social worker and social services home care workers, Crossroads care service, voluntary care workers, Marie Curie nurses and agency nurses, in addition to the patient and family.

Most people with MND prefer and expect to be cared for in their own home and the community team enable this to happen. As the disease progresses, constant review of the input of care will ensure that the required level of service is maintained.

Assessment centre

Some regional health authorities provide specialist assessment units whose role will be discussed later. The team may include the consultant, ward doctor, nurses, occupational therapist, physiotherapist, speech and language therapist, dietitian, technician/rehabilitation engineer, orthotist and social worker (see Chapter 4).

Hospital

The hospital team is usually only involved in the care of a person with MND if they require treatment for a condition secondary to their original diagnosis This may take the form of surgery, for example to perform a gastrostomy, or a medical condition such as renal colic or severe infection.

If an admission to hospital is necessary, the staff will need to be aware of the special requirements of a person with MND – diet, transfers, any special equipment and medication. Most carers are willing to help and advise staff, especially if direct communication with the patient is difficult (see p. 126).

Nursing/residential home

Whilst most people would prefer to receive care in their own homes, situations may occur which make this impossible. Few, if any, health authorities offer residential facilities for people with MND, so organization of residential care falls to the individual or family. Grants from the local social services department may help towards the cost of such care and a social worker may be approached to provide a list of registered homes within the area.

Following the introduction of the NHS and Community Care Act in April 1993, people who require nursing care as a result of a chronic medical condition may be entitled to financial help through care management services. The level of financial help available is dependent on the amount of savings held by the individual and requires assessment by a care manager who can be contacted directly or through a social worker.

Residential homes rarely employ trained nursing staff and their staff/client ratio is usually lower than that found in nursing homes. People with MND have ever-growing care needs and most residential homes recognize that they are not sufficiently well staffed to meet these needs, as the disease progresses.

Nursing homes employ trained nursing staff in addition to care attendants. Many nursing homes are large converted Victorian houses and may be unable to provide free movement for severely disabled residents in wheelchairs. Increasingly, purpose-built nursing homes are being opened which are able to accommodate people with MND; however, many younger people are reluctant to move to a nursing home as most of the residents are elderly.

Few nursing homes employ their own paramedical staff, but can organize physiotherapy and chiropody services where required if residents agree to fund this themselves. Community occupational therapists and speech and language therapists will usually advise on equipment which may be needed without direct charge, but will expect the home or individual to fund any items of equipment necessary, since few community loans departments issue equipment to nursing homes.

Hospice/palliative care unit

A hospice is a team or community concerned with enhancing the quality of remaining life for a patient and family struggling with mortal illness.

(Saunders, 1990).

Hospices and palliative care units undertake palliative and terminal care. Most hospices are charitably funded whilst palliative care units are funded by the National Health Service. Unfortunately, not all hospices or palliative care units are able to offer care to people with MND but the number that are willing is increasing. Few hospices are able to offer long-term residential care but may be able to offer respite care, symptom control, day care and home care support. The hospice team usually comprises a consultant, ward doctor, nurses, care assistants, physiotherapist, occupational therapist, Macmillan nurses, spiritual adviser and social worker. The services of other disciplines, such as speech and language therapists and dietitians, can be acquired as necessary.

TEAM FUNCTION

Direction

By definition, a team of people work together to achieve a common goal for all team members, as happens in most team sports. When working with a person with MND and their family, however, the team work together to achieve maximum effect for a small number of team members. Success is none the less important to each member of the team working in this situation, even if their involvement has been minimal.

Motivation

Health professionals usually work with a mixed client group. Working with people suffering from a progressive neurological condition such as MND is an area that is unfamiliar to some people and may not be one that they would choose. Whilst the work can be arduous, it can also be stimulating and rewarding if approached with a positive attitude. Problems need to be viewed as challenges rather than inconveniences.

Selection of the team

Staff selection is a skilled task which can be employed when building a team within a unit or hospital ward. When working in the community, individuals may be allocated to a case in a much more random manner. Allocation may depend on where the client lives or who has a space within their caseload at the time.

However the team is selected, it will function best if there is a member who has some experience of working with people who have MND. If this is not possible, someone within the team should be responsible for finding out about the disease, and both the physical and psychological problems which may arise.

Communication

Good communication between the team members is vital. Where the team operates from a unit or ward, weekly case reviews are usual, but updates will need to be more frequent if new information is received or the situation changes. Teams working in the community may find regular case conferences are too time consuming so may choose to communicate by telephone, meeting together less frequently.

The number of people working to support a person with MND and their family can be extensive and in the later stages of the illness, the situation can change considerably within a short space of time. Information, however insignificant it may seem, needs to be communicated to other members of the team promptly (see p. 34). The use of a keyworker to co-ordinate input of services is invaluable and will be discussed later in this chapter (p. 26).

Boundaries

Team members are people first and foremost, who have undertaken training for a professional qualification. Each one brings individual qualities and approaches to their work, which make them unique. In order that the team may function well, there will need to be a certain flexibility and generosity of spirit between team members as regards their individual professional boundaries.

There will be obvious core areas where each professional will operate, such as doctors prescribing medication, social workers advising on benefits and occupational therapists providing equipment to aid with daily living. Where team members receive requests outside their area of competence, they should feel able to hand over or share these areas of care with the appropriate team member.

There will, however, be other areas, for example psychological support, which are not quite so well defined. Providing support for the family is a task which usually falls to the team member with whom the patient feels comfortable discussing the issue concerned. Whilst confidentiality must be observed, it is important that team members be kept informed of the issues under discussion in an attempt to minimize collusion.

Health professionals working in this area need to be flexible and will gain experience and support from working in co-operation with each other.

Overlap of roles

Where health professionals are members of a multidisciplinary team working with people who have MND, there will need to be overlap of roles. This can be beneficial to the patient as it reduces the number of visits and intrusions on their time but it can cause identity problems for the health professional. Maintaining a core responsibility can enable the health professional to share peripheral issues more freely.

Team leader

A good team requires good leadership. A team leader has three overlapping areas of concern which must be kept in balance: achieving the task, building the team and developing individuals.

(Kaye, 1991)

It is usual for the general practitioner or medical director to be the leader of the team, since ultimate medical responsibility rests with him or her. This does not, however, mean that they should be placed in the position of making every decision, nor does it necessitate their undertaking the role of the keyworker (discussed later in this chapter). Individual members of the team need to be able to make decisions in their own field and where a team decision is required, discussions with other team members will often be necessary before settling on a final solution.

DISSENSION WITHIN THE TEAM

Problems in this area may be caused by the patient, family member or health professional. It is important to identify the problem and address it as soon as possible, if care of the patient is not to be disrupted.

Patient/family

Living with a progressive muscle wasting disease or caring for someone in that position is exhausting both emotionally and physically. Life changes cause stress to all members of the family and whilst help and support are vital it is, as yet, impossible to remove the ultimate cause of the stress and make the patient well again. The illness can continue for many months or years and, over that time, the pressures and stresses increase.

Problems, when they arise, are usually the result of conflict between the patient or family member and one or more members of the team. Most people with MND and their carers have definite views on the type of care they or their relative should receive and most disagreements occur when the views of the patient or family and those of the team member/s are at variance. Conflict may also occur if the type of care requested by the patient or their family is not available or only available from the private sector.

Care planning with the patient and carer can help to prevent this type of problem. If the team and patient/family agree on the type and amount of care necessary at the start and are involved as alterations are made, contention can be kept to a minimum. Good communication is essential to promote an effective working relationship and reduce conflict.

Health professionals

As has been stated, working in a multidisciplinary team requires flexibility and a willingness to share in the care of the patient. Conflict can occur when a team member is unwilling to pass on or share the responsibility of care when necessary. This is usually the result of a poor understanding of working as part of a multidisciplinary team and a more experienced member of the same profession may need to discuss the problem with the team member in an effort to resolve the situation.

Working with people with MND over a prolonged period of time can be stressful. There may be differences of opinion between team members as to the best course of action. Time should be given for the team to discuss these differences and finding the most acceptable solution may not be easy. The overriding consideration has to be the best interest of the patient but this must also fit in with the abilities of the family and the resources available to the multidisciplinary team.

Authority issues

In recent years, emphasis has been placed on the autonomy of the individual. Patient-centred care has grown from this way of thinking and has, together with an increased emphasis on community care, given patients much greater freedom of choice in the support and treatment they receive.

On occasions it may still be necessary for the medical practitioner to advise a course of action which they see to be medically correct, but with which the family are unhappy. This may occur in many different situations, examples being where admission to hospital is advised or where the administration of medication (particularly antibiotics in the terminal stage of the illness) is an issue.

Conflict of this sort can often be resolved by good communication and is made easier if the patient and family have a good working relationship with the medical practitioner. It is, however, impossible for the medical practitioner to force the patient or family into taking action unless it is their wish.

Authority can also cause conflict between health professionals within the team. A member of the team may see a situation developing within the family and feel that a specific course of action should be taken before the patient or family has agreed to accept this course of action. Once again, it is not possible to force the patient or family into acceptance of anything unless they are in agreement, but good communication between health professionals will usually enable a compromise to be reached.

TEAM MEMBERS

The team of people caring for a person with MND and the family can be large and will usually involve some, if not all, of the following personnel.

Patient and carer

The patient and carer are central members of the team. They should be involved in all decision making regarding treatment and input of care such that the provision of care is a partnership between the patient, the family and the team of people co-ordinating and providing the care.

In order that this can be achieved, the patient and carer will need access to information about the illness and resources available. They will also require time from various team members to discuss different options so that they may choose the most suitable course of action.

Each person is unique and the effects of MND are unpredictable, resulting in differing amounts of help being needed as time and the disease progress. The patient and carer will need a high level of support from the team to succeed in their efforts to identify and obtain the level of care appropriate to their needs.

General practitioner

Family doctors will usually be the first people with whom the patient and carer have contact since they will usually have arranged for neurological tests to confirm the diagnosis. Often the general practitioner will have known the patient and family for some time and will be well placed to offer help.

In addition to advising on the control of unpleasant symptoms, it will be necessary for the general practitioner to enlist the help of other health professionals. Physiotherapists need a medical referral before they can assess and treat patients. Occupational therapists and speech and language therapists may be contacted directly by the patient if desired, but referral by a medical practitioner will provide relevant information for the therapist before contact is made with the patient.

MND is an uncommon disease. Cochrane (1987) suggests that statistically, an average general practitioner can expect to see a new case of MND once in 26 years. It may, therefore, be necessary for the general practitioner to seek advice regarding certain areas of treatment or management from other team members or medical practitioners more experienced in the care of people with MND.

Consultant

Most people will have had their diagnosis confirmed by a neurologist. In some areas, the neurologist maintains contact with the patient through the illness and can be helpful in offering advice on control of symptoms specific to MND.

Where the neurologist feels unable to offer continuing care, support will be needed from elsewhere. Failure to identify additional support can result in feelings of isolation and abandonment within the patient and family. Once the diagnosis has been confirmed, future treatment involves palliation of unpleasant symptoms and co-ordination of support services. Consideration should be given to involving the palliative care consultant to supervise symptom control and subsequent management of care.

In any event, as the illness progresses and the patient becomes less mobile, travelling long distances for neurological appointments may become more difficult. Transfer of care to a local consultant, conversant with symptoms that can occur in the later stages of the illness, should then be considered, to ensure adequate treatment and support for the patient and their family during the final stages of the illness.

Nurses

Nursing may be undertaken by any or all of the following:

1. district nurse;
2. private or agency nurse;
3. nurses in hospital, hospice or nursing home;
4. Macmillan nurses.

District nurses

District nurses work within general practice. They can offer nursing care within the home which may include help with personal care, dressings, medication and bowel care. Their aim is to help the family to maintain the patient within the community.

Private or agency nurses

These can be employed to help with care of a person within their own home. They can be employed through an agency or by private arrangement with the person concerned. Cost varies depending on the degree of training, the number of hours worked and when the hours are worked (day or night). Funding for the cost of a private nurse rests with the individual and their family unless financial assistance can be obtained. A social worker can advise on the likelihood of help in meeting this cost.

Nurses in hospital, hospice or nursing home

It may be necessary, on occasion, for a person to be admitted to a residential establishment for treatment or respite care. It is important that the nurses and care staff are informed of the regime of care at home, so they can maintain continuity as far as possible whilst the patient is in their care. It can be helpful to provide written care plans for reference by staff involved in the care of the patient.

Most people wish to remain at home and most carers hope that this will be possible. As time and the disease progress, it may become necessary, despite support, for care to be transferred permanently to a residential home. The transition from home to residential care can be eased if the patient has visited the future home previously.

Macmillan nurses

In some areas, Macmillan nurses are prepared to become involved in the care of people with MND. Macmillan nurses are registered general nurses with a district nurse qualification who have undertaken further English Nursing Board training in care of the dying. They can be a useful source of advice on symptom control, particularly in the later stages of the disease, but they do not undertake 'hands on' nursing duties.

Physiotherapist

Physiotherapists work as part of the rehabilitation team in hospitals, health centres and, in some areas, they visit people in their own homes. They can help to maintain functional independence and mobility for as long as possible. As mobility deteriorates, they can teach active-assisted and passive movements to keep joints mobile and decrease aching of the joints. Chest care, breathing exercises, splinting, relaxation and transfer techniques are other areas in which the physiotherapist may be able to offer help and advice.

The physiotherapist will need a letter of referral from a medical practitioner (general practitioner or hospital consultant) before beginning treatment, and their involvement should continue throughout the course of the illness. Early referral to the physiotherapist will enable her to provide the best service to the patient and family (see also Chapter 4).

Occupational therapist

Referral to an occupational therapist is often made soon after, or in some cases just before, diagnosis. The initial symptoms of the disease are usually such that they prevent the person from carrying out some activities of daily living. The occupational therapist has much to offer since provision of equipment, problem-solving advice and energy-saving techniques can encourage and increase independence. The philosophy of occupational therapy and its holistic approach can also help to reinforce and improve self-esteem.

The occupational therapist can advise on equipment available to ease problems of daily living, seating, pressure relief, wheelchairs, environmental control systems and adaptations (such as ramps or building alterations) which may be necessary to the home. They may also be able to advise on holidays and leisure activities available in the area.

Referral to a community occupational therapist can come directly from the patient or family, but hospital-based occupational therapists need a referral from a medical practitioner. In any event, a full medical and social history from a medical practitioner will need to be sought, to facilitate assessment and planning future care. Early involvement of the occupational therapist is recommended to maximize independence and ensure that any alterations to the home can be actioned in good time (see also Chapter 4).

Speech and language therapist

Speech and language therapists specialize in helping people who have speech and/or swallowing difficulties. They can offer much help and advice to the person with MND and the family. Speech and language therapists work from hospitals or health centres and in some areas will visit people in their own homes if travelling is difficult. Contact with the speech and language therapist can be made through the general practitioner or direct contact can be made by the patient or their carer.

Speech is the most common method of communication used by people in everyday life. Whilst it is possible to communicate in other ways, speech is the quickest and most effective. It is helpful to both the therapist and patient if referrals are made at an early stage as this gives time for relationships to be developed whilst speech is still intelligible. If speech deteriorates, the speech and language therapist can advise on the most appropriate method of alternative communication.

Eating and drinking may become difficult as the disease progresses. Speech and language therapists can advise on the best food textures, positioning for eating and methods of stimulating swallowing. Speech and language therapy involvement, once begun, will last through the course of the illness. It should be possible, with thought, to ensure that some form of communication, however basic, can continue despite the severity of the disease (see also Chapters 4 and 6).

Dietitian

Dietitians are located in most district general hospitals. Their help may be necessary if swallowing becomes difficult and advice is needed to maintain adequate nutrition. The dietitian works closely with the speech and language therapist and in some areas, their roles may overlap.

Referral can be made by a general practitioner or hospital consultant and may necessitate a visit to an out-patient clinic. Where this causes problems, it may be possible for the dietitian to visit the patient at home.

If swallowing problems become very severe, thought may need to be given to alternative methods of obtaining adequate nutrition and fluids. If parenteral feeding such as a naso-gastric tube or gastrostomy becomes necessary, the dietitian will advise on the liquid feeds available (see also Chapters 4 and 6).

Social worker

Social workers are employed by the local social services department and may be found in the local area office or in a hospital department. They can provide advice on benefits, housing, services to help the patient and family or advice on holidays for the disabled.

Referral can be made by the patient or family directly to the area office, if contact has not been made through the hospital. Social workers can be a great support to people living with this type of disease and should be contacted as soon as possible after diagnosis.

Care manager

The NHS and Community Care Act implemented in 1993 recognized the individual's need for appropriate care. This care may be in the patient's own home or in a residential setting, depending on the needs of the patient. Care managers ensure that an individual's need for care is met and that where the patient's funds are insufficient, funding in full or part is available to enable this to happen.

People with MND usually need a high level of care during the course of their illness and a care manager may need to be involved to ensure that these needs are addressed. Assessments from health professionals working with the patient are usually sought and a meeting is arranged with the patient, carer, care manager and health professionals to work out the most efficient way to provide the care needed.

Once the care package is in place, the care manager usually withdraws from the team until the patient's needs change and alterations need to be made to the care package.

Religious support

Religious belief is the way that many people in our society express their spirituality. Some people are regular members of a religious faith, although many more express a belief in God but do not have a regular commitment to a particular faith. Most hospitals have a full-time or part-time chaplain who will be willing to talk about spiritual issues.

There are many people who find difficulty in verbalizing spiritual issues. Set religious offices such as communion and meditation can be a way of meeting these needs. It has also been found that readings from the Gospels hold special significance and people may identify these with their own needs. It is important that people are able to contact a chaplain or priest if they feel the need, whether or not they have an established faith.

Voluntary care organizations

Many areas have voluntary agencies who can offer help and support to people with MND and their families. Information can be obtained from the local social services office or from the general practitioner. Their role is usually to work alongside the statutory services provided by social services or the health authority in an attempt to widen the area of care available.

Referral to these services may need to come from a health professional and should be made early, since many have a waiting list for their help.

Motor Neurone Disease Association (MNDA)

The role of the MNDA is outlined in more detail later in the book (Appendix A), but members of the organization usually form part of the multidisciplinary team. The regional care adviser, local branch or the helpline can provide help and support to people with MND and their families.

THE ROLE OF THE KEYWORKER

As has been stated, a large number of people can be involved in the team. A keyworker can ensure that the team is achieving its aim and that the patient and family are receiving the best care possible. The role of the keyworker can be summarized as follows.

Communication with the family

The keyworker can only remain effective if she can communicate well with the patient and family. People with MND are often reluctant to admit to problems they are facing and unless they are encouraged to discuss these difficulties, will resist help. Whoever undertakes the role of the keyworker will need to develop and maintain a relationship of trust with the patient and family throughout the course of the illness.

Knowledge of the disease

It will be necessary for the keyworker to increase her knowledge of the disease. It is likely that the patient and/or family will wish to know as much as possible about the illness and will ask the keyworker as the most easily accessible and approachable person. Knowledge of the possible progression of the illness will help the keyworker to explore potentially difficult areas in an effort to avert a crisis.

Preservation of privacy

Many people with MND resent the quantity of helpers needed to maintain care within the home. This can be distressing to the whole family and cause great friction between different family members. The keyworker can co-ordinate visits and calls by health professionals and so maintain as much privacy as possible for the family.

Involvement of other health professionals

Ensuring that representatives of the various health professions are involved appropriately falls to the keyworker; confusion can exist in this area if no one takes responsibility for the task. Poor care management will result if team members are unaware that their services are needed, and the patient may suffer unnecessarily.

Co-ordination of information and care between different teams

Where a patient is moving between the community and hospital or residential care, the keyworker can liaise between the teams and ensure that information about the patient's care is communicated, effecting a smooth transfer.

Education

MND is a comparatively rare condition. Few people have in-depth knowledge of the probable disease progression or management of people with the illness. If this is the case, it is important for the team to find out as much information as possible.

The keyworker may need to share her knowledge of the disease with other members of the team. Health professionals working in a community team may not have worked together before and may have little experience of the restrictions that MND can place on the patient and family. Building up knowledge about the disease can also help in the future, where individual team members may be working with other patients who have MND.

The MNDA publish a series of booklets about the disease and the roles of different health professionals. Contact with the MNDA regional care adviser and the local branch in a given area (details from MNDA National Office) can provide information regarding available help.

STAFF SUPPORT

Working with people who are living with a progressively disabling illness over a comparatively long period of time can cause stress. It is foolish to overlook this fact, so thought should be given to the type of support needed by team members. There are few firm thoughts on this subject; what follows are ideas which may prove helpful.

Support from within the team

Individual team members experience stress as a result of different situations and may need help to overcome their difficulties. Many situations cause stress, the most notable being a sudden deterioration in the patient's condition or a crisis within the family requiring extra input from one or more team member. Support is usually needed at the time or immediately after an incident occurs and any team member may be approached for help.

Emotions within the family are often intense and it is not unusual for any team member working in this situation to have to deal with anger, profound sadness and distress from the patient or family. The resulting exhaustion can be reduced if the health professionals can discuss their feelings with other team members, and gain reassurance that the event was handled as well as possible.

Support networks of this nature are usually naturally occurring, as some team members will relate together better than others. It can be helpful for the keyworker to check within the team that everyone has access to a person with whom they can discuss matters of this kind.

External support

Social workers and counsellors, because of the nature of their work, have time set aside for supervision. This enables them to have a period of time each week to discuss cases with a fellow member of the professional team who is not involved directly with any of the clients.

This is rarely found in other health professions but it is an option which can be adopted by others, if they are prepared to set this up for themselves. Most health authorities and many general practices have counselling services which may be accessed by employees. Alternatively, private counselling may be sought if it is thought necessary, but the cost of this would have to be met by the individual.

Positive feedback

It is important to acknowledge when achievements are made. Problems and difficulties often overshadow accomplishments which may then be overlooked. Achievements can include funding sought and found for a holiday, a piece of equipment obtained or a member of the team who has helped the family through a particularly difficult time. Appropriate praise can help to dissipate stress.

Relaxation

Working with people who have life-threatening illnesses can cause exhaustion if emotional expenditure exceeds income. Consideration of emotional recreation may include social interests outside work, exercise, individual beliefs or philosophies and personal time to express emotions. It is important that individual team members recognize their own limitations and develop the ability to care for themselves, in addition to caring for others.

CONCLUSION

In this chapter it has been shown that teamwork is essential in the care of people with MND. Promotion of good team function has been discussed and thought has been given to areas where difficulties may arise. Teams and team members have been identified and the role of the keyworker in this type of work has been discussed. Finally, some ideas on staff support have been suggested to enable the team to continue to function at the best level possible throughout its involvement with the patient and family.

REFERENCES

Cassidy, S. (1988) *Sharing the Darkness*, Darton, Longman and Todd, London.

Cochrane, G. (1987) *The Management of Motor Neurone Disease*, Churchill Livingstone, Edinburgh.

Gibran, K. (1991) *The Prophet*, Pan Books, London (first published 1926).

Kaye, P. (1991) *Symptom Control in Hospice and Palliative Care* (revised edn), Hospice Education Institute, Connecticut, USA.

Saunders, C. (1990) *Hospice and Palliative Care – An Interdisciplinary Approach*, Edward Arnold, London.

FURTHER READING

Burnard, P. (1989) *Counselling Skills for Health Professionals*, Chapman & Hall, London.

Dunlop, R. J. and Hockley, J. M. (1990) *Terminal Care Support Teams*, Oxford University Press, Oxford.

Hull, R., Ellis, M. and Sargent, V. (1989) *Teamwork in Palliative Care*, Radcliffe Medical Press, Oxford.

Robbins, J. (1989) *Caring for the Dying Patient and the Family*, Harper and Row, New York.

Stewart, W. (1985) *Counselling in Rehabilitation*, Croom Helm, London.

Turner, A., Foster, M., and Johnson, S. (eds) (1992) *Occupational Therapy and Physical Dysfunction*, Churchill Livingstone, Edinburgh.

3 | Aims and objectives of the multidisciplinary team

Theory is the lens through which we see reality more clearly.

(Keilhofner, 1985).

INTRODUCTION

Keilhofner, together with Burke and Igi, devised and developed the Model of Human Occupation during the 1970s and 1980s. It is widely used by occupational therapists to order assessment and thinking, providing a link between the Human Occupations/Activities Theory and occupational therapy practice.

A team remains effective as long as it formulates and follows clear aims and objectives. In order that this may be achieved, it will require relation to a frame or frames of reference which can be defined as 'an organised body of knowledge, principles and research findings which forms the conceptual basis of **a particular aspect** of practice. It is based on cognitive, perceptual, psychological and social considerations and is used to explain the relationship between theory and practice' (Foster, in Turner, Foster and Johnson, 1992).

Each profession has specific frames of reference which form the foundation to its practice and these individual frames of reference should interrelate, as does the multidisciplinary team. The frame of reference suggested here, based on humanistic theory, can form a basis for intervention by individual members of the team.

Maslow and Rogers are the most well known humanistic psychologists. Their work is founded around the importance of the individual (self-concept) and the belief in the basic ability of the individual to grow and develop towards their own potential, a state they call 'self-actualization'. The individual is central to their thinking, possesses a basic goodness and contains forces that direct growth and development to full potential, unless blocked or distorted by environmental conditions.

PHILOSOPHY OF CARE

The philosophy of care found to be most effective reflects this frame of reference and is most closely aligned to that of the hospice movement. The ideals set out present a challenge to the health professional but, if considered and implemented, will result in good quality care being delivered.

Hospice philosophy embraces the humanistic theory put forward by Maslow (1970) and Rogers (1967) but also acknowledges a spirituality within the individual. It is based on patient- and family-centred care, recognition of the needs of the individual, good communication, multidisciplinary teamwork, staff support and bereavement aftercare. St Christopher's Hospice in Sydenham, London, was opened in 1967 and with it, views and ideas on palliative care began to unfold, which have and are still slowly changing attitudes towards the care of people suffering from life-threatening diseases.

The role of the hospice and palliative care unit has developed rapidly over the past 25 years and as with every community, continues to grow and evolve in line with the needs of its consumers. In some instances, it would be inappropriate to introduce a person who has been newly diagnosed with MND to their local hospice or palliative care unit. That said, other people have gained great support from out-patient appointments with the palliative care consultant, and the knowledge that there are facilities to care for them as their condition worsens. In addition, it has been found that hospice philosophy (summarized below) can be applied to the continuing care of these people throughout their illness, in a form modified to suit their needs.

Patient- and family-centred care

Throughout adult life, decisions have to be made. These may be comparatively minor – for example, the choice of food for a meal; alternatively they may be more significant – choosing a career or a partner. By making and carrying out decisions, people effect control over their lives to a greater or lesser extent.

Whilst a person with MND is able to make decisions, they are progressively more reliant upon others for their wishes to be carried out. It can be very difficult to remember that whilst patients may be immobile and have difficulty communicating, their intellect is as sharp as ever.

Usually, the patient and carer are best placed to know their own needs.

Time should be taken to discuss their wishes and, if at all possible, these wishes should be implemented. There will be occasions when this is not possible because of a lack of resources or the facilities required. If this is the case, time needs to be given to discussing alternatives with the patient and carer so that they can choose a modified plan of action.

It is rare to find a person with MND who perceives himself as being ill. People with MND rarely feel unwell unless they have a secondary infection or uncontrolled symptoms and they do not easily fit themselves into the concept which society holds of a disabled person.

MND does not only affect the person with the illness; as one carer commented, 'I feel more paralysed by this disease than my husband'. People do not live in isolation and since the person with the disease needs progressively more help to function, it often happens that a close family member becomes the main carer. Other family members may also become involved in caring from time to time. Individual carers have their own limitations and will need help and support to provide the level of care necessary, particularly if the person with MND wishes to be cared for at home over an extended period of time.

MND is a neurological condition but, because of the rate of progression of the disease, the person can become terminally ill in a comparatively short space of time. This will require a philosophy of care that can be applied to each stage during the progression of the disease. This illness can be arduous for the individual and carer alike, but by working with the family as a whole, it is possible to provide a care package to meet their needs.

Recognition of the needs of the individual

People have basic needs which can be identified as physical, psychological, emotional and spiritual. They are interconnected and need to be balanced to allow a person to remain healthy. Identification of physical, emotional and psychological needs is relatively easy and most health professionals feel quite comfortable assisting in meeting these needs.

Spirituality is an area of need that is often neglected. The reason for this may be in part that, in our culture, low priority is attached to spiritual needs until a crisis develops. A crisis brings life into sharp focus and necessitates consideration of spiritual issues.

'Man is not destroyed by suffering. He is destroyed by suffering without meaning' (Frankl, 1953). Living with MND challenges many people to search for meaning within their lives and they may require the help and support of a companion in the task.

Religion can be one way for a person to explore and express spirituality. David Langford (Free Church chaplain to Moorgreen Hospital,

Southampton) defines the difference between spiritual and religious matters thus:

> Spiritual relates to a concern with ultimate issues and life principles and is often seen as a search for meaning in a person's life. Religious is the practical expression of spirituality through a framework of beliefs often actively pursued in rituals and religious practice.
>
> *(Langford, 1989).*

The search for meaning may be expressed through questions such as 'Why me?' or 'What have I done to deserve this?'. These questions in themselves do not have answers but they are often an indication that the person wishes to talk and try to make sense of a particular situation.

It is important to respect individual religious beliefs and not to share one's own unless asked; even then, caution should be observed. People who are facing life-threatening situations can feel very vulnerable and highly pressured by dogmatic religious views.

People travelling on a spiritual journey, particularly when trying to make sense of an illness like MND, will choose a person with whom they feel comfortable to discuss these issues. It is important to remember, however, that not all health professionals feel comfortable discussing such matters and, if this is the case, it may be necessary to find someone who will be able to offer help in this area.

The person to whom this task falls must be able to offer both time and patience: time to listen and understand and patience to stay with the individual even in despair and distress. A helper cannot provide the answers but, by creating an environment where questions are discussed openly, can help patients to find answers within themselves. More important to individuals is the knowledge that however difficult life may become, they will not be deserted, even if the situation appears bleak.

Symptom control

MND is incurable at present but it is not untreatable. Any unpleasant symptoms that are experienced need careful assessment and treatment, where necessary, by medication or alterations to the management plan. This should be undertaken by a medical practitioner conversant with the needs of this patient group.

Communication

This skill does not come easily to some people but can be learned. The basis of good communication lies in the ability to listen and understand what is being said, and to respond in an appropriate way. Good communication also involves eliciting relevant information. Asking the right questions and clarifying the answers, rather than working on assumptions, will often prevent misunderstandings.

Many people do not communicate easily. When faced with a crisis in their lives, they need to learn to communicate in order to resolve the crisis. One carer explained, 'I find it very difficult to talk about how I feel – I would much rather go and hang wallpaper or do something practical'. People used to dealing with life on a practical level can experience difficulty in giving thought to more abstract issues.

There is an added dimension to communication when working with a patient with MND. As the disease progresses, it is possible that speech will become affected. In 1981, Saunders, Walsh and Smith found that in their sample of 100 people with MND, 90% became dysarthric and of these, 80% developed unintelligible speech prior to death. Despite this, it is important to maintain communication with patients if that is their wish, however basic a form this may take. Good communication also extends to members of the multidisciplinary team (p.17).

Teamwork

Teamwork is discussed in some detail in Chapter 2. The main importance to the philosophy of care are the benefits to the patient of multiprofessional expertise in handling different problems.

Staff support

Staff support has been discussed in Chapter 2, but forms an integral part of this philosophy of care.

Bereavement support

Part of care of the dying is care of the bereaved: they are two sides of the same coin.

(Lamerton, 1980).

Grieving is a normal, healing process and can be experienced by anyone following the death of someone close to them. It begins when the person is told that they will not live as long as they had originally hoped and involves the person concerned and those to whom they are close.

Consideration should be given to this through the progression of the illness and for the family after the death of the patient. Bereavement support is discussed in more detail in Chapter 8.

THEORETICAL FRAMEWORK

Humanistic theory recognizes the individual as a 'whole' being who is essentially good and has the power to change given certain circumstances.

In 1954, Abraham Maslow (1908–70) put forward the theory that people are motivated by a series of needs which he subdivided into those that ensure survival and those that enable a person to develop to full potential. Maslow's hierarchy of needs can be represented by a diagrammatic pyramid which emphasizes that the needs lower down on the pyramid must be satisfied, at least in part, before the person can consider those at a higher level (Figure 3.1).

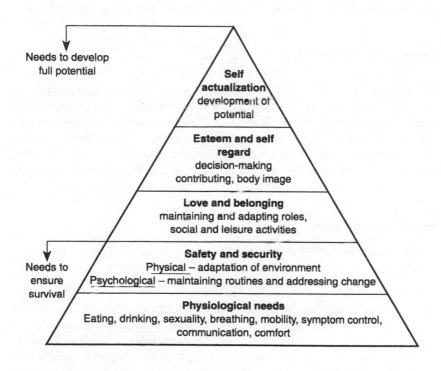

Figure 3.1 Maslow's hierarchy of needs as applied to people with MND.

The fundamental needs are those associated with survival: food, drink, air to breathe and other basic requirements of life. If those needs are met, people then need to feel safe and secure from danger and if this is met, their social needs – for love and acceptance by friends – can be addressed. Following this is a need to feel good about oneself and finally, if all the lower levels are at least partially satisfied, a person can consider developing their potential as an individual. Maslow refers to this as 'self-actualization'. An illustration of this could be that a person is unlikely to want to read a book or engage in some other activity to broaden the mind while experiencing constant discomfort or pain.

Carl Rogers (1902–87) believed that people had two important psychological needs: the first, to fulfil their true potential; the second, a need for positive regard from others. If these two needs were met, it enabled an individual to develop a healthy personality. In this way, if the health professional has a relationship with the patient in which the patient feels valued for himself, not needing to seek approval from the therapist, he will be encouraged to make decisions and develop his life.

In order to plan patient care, aims and objectives can be related to the philosophy of care. To ensure that these aims and objectives are met, specific goals can then be made related to Maslow's hierarchy of needs.

AIMS AND OBJECTIVES

Aims and objectives should be common to the entire multidisciplinary team, whilst specific goals will usually be set by individual team members. On occasion, two workers from different professions may be working towards the same goal but may approach the task in different ways. Where a team work together regularly, their aims will usually coincide but when working with a team of people drawn from different areas, it may be necessary to clarify aims to ensure that the team is working towards the same ends.

Improve quality of life

You matter because you are you. You matter to the last moment of your life . . .

(Saunders cited in Zora and Zora, 1981).

The physical impact of MND on a person's life often starts to become apparent before the diagnosis is confirmed. Becoming progressively less able to perform simple tasks related to daily living requires action to restore independence, where possible, by use of equipment or compensatory techniques. Attention to unpleasant symptoms, methods of communication, mobility, productivity and adequate nutritional intake can all improve the quality of a person's life.

Encourage internal locus of control

Individuals who see control as lying within their own realm of responsibility are more likely to contribute their own ideas and to be more evaluative about others' suggestions.

(Foster, in Turner, Foster and Johnson, 1992).

Individuals have varying ideas as to whether they have control over their own lives or whether their lives are controlled by other forces. Helping to maintain roles, routines and customs and encouraging active participation in their treatment can encourage patients to retain or regain control over their lives. If it is no longer possible to maintain existing roles, thought should be given to changing or adapting roles or delegating functions within existing roles. Change needs to be introduced slowly to reduce feelings of insecurity.

People who are ill often feel that they have little control over their lives. In this situation, offering advice requires thought since it is rarely welcomed unless requested. Patients and their families can be overwhelmed by too many suggestions of ways in which their lives may be improved, leaving them feeling powerless and out of control.

Patient/family-centred care

Loneliness is not so much a matter of being alone as of not belonging. Everyone needs person to person contact ... I rarely feel lonely because although I am alone for many hours I always have the feeling of belonging.

(Holden, 1980).

Establishing the patient and family within the team reinforces feelings of belonging, as does encouragement to build and continue relationships.

As has been stated, people are often reluctant to admit to difficulties they are experiencing and may need help to do this. There may also be fears and anxieties about the present and the future which, if not acknowledged, may become overwhelming and lead to feelings of isolation.

Promotion of self-esteem

The client not only accepts himself – a phrase which may carry the connotation of a grudging and reluctant acceptance of the inevitable – he actually comes to *like* himself. This is not a bragging or self-assertive liking; it is rather a quiet pleasure in being one's self.

(Rogers, 1967).

An illness like MND changes people's perception of themselves both physically and psychologically. It is, however, possible for the person to continue, or become able, to like themselves. This does require effort on the part of the health professionals in the attitude and esteem in which they hold the individual.

Self-acceptance is helped, at least in part, by the courage and determination that most people with this disease demonstrate, illustrated by Saunders, Walsh and Smith (1981): '... The recent comment of a neurologist visiting the Hospice, "A most dreadful disease!" was countered by a nursing auxiliary who has worked here for ten years, "But they are such splendid people" '.

Development of potential

Developing potential is '. . . The primary motivation for creativity as the organism forms new relationships to the environment in its endeavour most fully to be itself . . .'

(Rogers, 1967).

MND progressively strips away physical and psychological irrelevancies. As the person becomes physically weaker, relationships become more important since expression in other ways becomes more difficult. Building a relationship on unconditional positive regard enables the health professional to help in the process of developing the potential of the patient.

Bereavement support

Grieving begins at the time of diagnosis and continues through the progression of the illness, death and bereavement. Whilst this is not addressed in Maslow's hierarchy of needs, it is none the less important for the patient and family. Efforts to help the family to function in a way appropriate to them during the progression of the illness usually help them to work through their grief after the death of the patient.

Bereavement support may be arranged as formal or informal support. For many people, informal support will be sufficient but it is important to know the agencies who could offer help should the need arise (see Chapter 8).

GOALS

Provision of care also requires setting of more specific aims for team members to work towards. Whilst the ultimate aim must be to provide an environment where the patient and their family can function and grow during the progression of the illness, someone will have to address themselves to the problem of enabling the patient to get out of bed each morning, and the specific problems this presents to the individual and family.

Specific goals will need to be reassessed at regular intervals as the illness progresses. For this reason, it is important to set realistic targets which are achievable. There may be occasions where hope is kept alive for the individual by the thought of a longer-term goal, such as a visit by a relative from some distance away or the birth of a child or grandchild. These longer-term goals should not be underestimated in their power to lift morale, and should not be set too far into the future if at all possible.

It should not be forgotten that as a member of the team, the patient will also wish to set his own goals. These may require the help of other members of the team if they are to be achieved.

Maslow's hierarchy of needs forms a framework for development of specific aims. In relating aims to a framework, it must be remembered that people are individuals and rarely fit neatly into categories. The following will hopefully provide a guide to the principles of care found to be effective when working with this patient group and their families.

Physiological needs

The need for basic elements of survival is, in Maslow's opinion, the fundamental necessity of the individual. Where possible, independence in attaining them is desirable. Independence is a subjective state, since areas that are important to one person will not necessarily be important to another. This should be borne in mind when setting targets. Short-term goals in this area might include the following elements.

- *Food and drink.* Ensuring the individual is able to consume sufficient food and drink to prevent him from becoming hungry and thirsty. Initially this may require provision of equipment to enable the patient to eat and drink independently, whilst later it may involve employment of a carer to ensure that this need is met.
- *Bodily functions.* Consideration of the individual's ability to wash and dress, get to the toilet, open bowels regularly.
- *Sexuality.* Sometimes an area of difficulty for people with a progressive physical illness. Many health professionals do not feel comfortable discussing this need with their patients. In some cases, discussion in this area would not be welcome but a general awareness of the existence of a person's sexuality can indicate a willingness to address the issue if the patient wishes.
- *Breathing.* Teaching relaxation techniques, visualization and breathing exercises can help reduce fear of suffocation. Medication may be used in addition to maximize lung function.
- *Communication.* Attention to maximizing speech and the assessment and provision of communication equipment as necessary.
- *Symptom control.* Consideration of medication and management techniques used in the treatment of unpleasant symptoms.
- *Mobility.* Provision of walking aids and wheelchairs, exercises and passive movements to maintain joint mobility and comfort.
- *Energy conservation.* Teaching energy-saving techniques can conserve energy to use on activities that are enjoyable. This may also involve provision of equipment to help with daily living.
- *Comfort.* Consideration of pressure relief when sitting or lying.

Safety and security

To encourage a stable environment in which the patient and family can function requires consideration of physical and psychological issues.

Physical

- *Adaptations.* Alterations to the home may be necessary to enable a person to be cared for in the community.
- *Environmental control systems.* These can provide increased control of the home environment despite disability.
- *Support for the carer.* This may take the form of day care, respite care or sitters to enable the carer to go out. Time set aside for the carer to voice their concerns and needs may also be necessary.

Psychological

- *Maintaining routines.* Visiting at times convenient to the patient and carer wherever possible.
- *Addressing change.* Discussing problems and working out, with patient and carer, a modified framework. Minimizing change where necessary to maximize security.
- *Activating change.* Where a change is necessary, e.g. a move from home to residential care, the patient and family will require support from members of the team.

Love and belonging

On the whole, people are sociable. They have a need to love and be loved. The patient may need help in maintaining his position in his social world as he faces a rather uncertain future. He may also need help in letting go and saying goodbye to friends and relatives.

- *Maintaining roles.* Taking time to discover the roles of the patient and carer within the family, and providing help where necessary to enable them to continue or adjust.
- Establish patient and family's place within the team.
- *Travelling.* The individual may need advice on car mobility, holiday venues and equipment needed.
- *Reminiscence.* Encouragement to think and talk about their lives. Consideration of family relationships and unfinished family business.
- *Facing the future.* Securing the future for spouse and children, help with business affairs, benefits, making a will, discussion of aspects of faith, planning the funeral.

- *Social and leisure activities.* Helping to maintain existing social interests where possible or adapting them to the current situation.

Esteem and self-regard

To live a full life, people need to feel good about themselves. Just as they need to love and be loved, they also need to contribute to life in whatever way they are able. If an opportunity is made for this to happen, self-esteem will grow.

- *Decision making.* Ensuring that individuals are as much a part of this as they have always been.
- *Body image.* Patients may need reassurance that they are still socially acceptable people.
- *Personal appearance.* Attention to personal care, make-up, hair care, nail care and clothing.
- *Ability to give.* This may be in the form of presents, writing, interviews about their lives or the illness, to help others. Many people with MND become experienced listeners as the following comment illustrates: 'People just drop in for a chat or to give me the latest ward news and dare I say it, even the occasional moan. Unless they are very good actors I have the feeling that mostly they come because they want to, which is very good for my ego' (Holden, 1980).
- *Giving to the family.* Preparation of a photograph album or scrap book.
- *Long-term decisions.* Participation in planning for the future of the family.

Self-actualization

To begin to develop his potential, a person must feel good about himself. Growing towards self-actualization is a continuing process rather than an end product. It may be, in reality, that a person experiences moments of passing fulfilment on the journey rather than achieving a permanent state of self-actualization. Ultimately, it is hoped that the person would be able to work through feelings surrounding his illness and be freed to live his life to the fullest extent of his capabilities.

As MND progresses, relationships are often the main outlet left to the person with the illness. It would follow, therefore, that the formulation of aims to help in this area would have to be of a psychological nature. Rogers (1967) suggests ways in which constructive creativity may be fostered. These will form the basis for these short-term goals and are, in effect, a basis for the therapeutic relationship.

- *Unconditional positive regard.* Acknowledgement that the patient is a worthwhile person in his own right and is intrinsically good.

- *Absence of external evaluation.* Adoption of a non-judgemental approach to the patient and their family.
- *Empathetic understanding.* Attempt to see the world as the patient or carer sees it and to move around within that world whilst maintaining a hold on one's own reality.
- *Psychological freedom.* To allow the person to be free and to assume responsibility for his own actions.

CONCLUSION

In this chapter, the use of a framework and philosophy of care is discussed. These are based on the humanistic approach to care and can be adapted for use wherever the patient is receiving treatment. Suggestions for aims and objectives and specific goals are put forward, related to humanistic theory and hospice philosophy.

REFERENCES

Frankl, V.E. (1953) *Man's Search for Meaning*, Hodder and Stoughton, London.
Holden, T. (1980) Patiently speaking. *Nursing Times*, June 12, 1035–6.
Keilhofner, G. (ed.) (1985) *The Model of Human Occupation*, Williams and Wilkins, Baltimore, USA.
Lamerton, R. (1980) *Care of the Dying* (revised edn), Penguin, Harmondsworth.
Langford, D. (1989) *Where is God in All This? A Study in the Spiritual Care of the Terminally Ill*, Countess Mountbatten House (Education), Southampton, England.
Maslow, A. (1970) *Motivation and Personality* (2nd edn), Harper and Row, London.
Rogers, C. (1967) *On Becoming A Person*, Constable, London.
Saunders, C., Walsh, T.D. and Smith, M. (1981) *Hospice – The Living Idea*, Edward Arnold, London.
Turner, A., Foster, M. and Johnson, S. (eds) (1992) *Occupational Therapy and Physical Dysfunction* (3rd edn), Churchill Livingstone, Edinburgh.
Zora, V. and Zora, R. (1981) *A Way to Die*, Sphere Books Ltd., London.

FURTHER READING

Atkinson, R., Smith, E., Bem, D. and Hilgard, E. R. (1993) *Introduction to Psychology* (11th edn), Harcourt Brace Jovanovich Publishers.
Fransella, F. (1982) *Psychology for Occupational Therapists*, Macmillan Publishing, London.
Gross, R. (1992) *Psychology* (2nd edn), Hodder and Stoughton, London.
Hayes, N. (1988) *A First Course in Psychology* (2nd edn), Nelson, Walton-on-Thames, Surrey.
Thorne, B. (1992) *Carl Rogers*, Sage Publications, London.

Assessment and treatment planning | 4

> Patients usually have many different problems. A full assessment demonstrates a serious intent to be in control of all the facts. The way it is done is a powerful message.
>
> *(Kaye, 1991).*

INTRODUCTION

Planning and implementation of treatment without full assessment of the needs of the individual will result in provision of inferior quality care. Resources will not be used efficiently and the cost, in both time and money, will be significantly increased. It is, therefore, surprising that very little has been published on assessment of the needs of people with MND.

A team approach to treatment requires a team approach to assessment. This can be easily addressed if the patient is being seen in an out-patient or hospital setting, but can be more difficult if, following diagnosis, the patient is discharged home immediately into the care of the community team.

The following chapter acknowledges that there are vast differences between management of the disease in different areas of the country, but tries to suggest ways in which assessment may be managed to provide a better standard of care for people with MND.

AIMS OF ASSESSMENT

> Assessment is a conscious task ... The process of assessment is not confined to the gathering of data, but is dependent upon its interpretation and evaluation.
>
> *(Foster in Turner, Foster and Johnson, 1992).*

Whoever performs an assessment must be constantly aware that the information they receive needs to be interpreted and evaluated. Observations and results, whilst interesting in their own right, cannot be considered of value as assessment material without explanation.

The overall aims of assessment are summarized in the following sections.

Gather information

A diagnosis of MND is usually reached following tests carried out by the neurologist. Once the diagnosis has been confirmed, the neurologist usually communicates the diagnosis to the patient and anyone that the patient wishes to have present. At this time it is important that the patient and family are assured of continued support by a senior medical practitioner conversant with their condition.

The neurologist may wish to continue supervision of care or may transfer care to another consultant if it is felt that this is more appropriate. Newrick and Langton-Hewer concluded from their study of 42 patients in 1984 that management of care of people with MND should be supervised by neurologists or by use of 'clinical assistants who had received appropriate training'. Following the move by more hospices to undertake care of people with MND, many palliative care consultants now have appropriate experience and understand the needs of this patient group.

Following diagnosis, an appointment with the appropriate consultant should be offered to the patient and member/s of the family. This time can be used to discuss issues arising from the diagnosis and can also be used to address the continuing care of the patient and family. The initial assessment is most important. Adequate time should be allowed at this interview to explore areas that are important to the patient and family. Questions can be asked at this time which would be difficult to ask at future interviews.

The consultant may wish to involve other members of the multidisciplinary team in the initial interview or may prefer to arrange for them to be seen separately. Information received and explanations given should be noted down for future reference. This can improve team communication, particularly when the consultant carries out the interview alone.

Each member of the team will have an interest in a different aspect of patient care, but they will all require basic information about relevant medical problems, home and social situation. General information should be communicated to each team member by the person who has the first contact with the patient. Whilst this will not prevent repetition it will help to keep it to a minimum. Information will be given and received throughout the course of the illness. Follow-up assessments will obviously be necessary for the purpose of review, as well as reinforcing the attempts of the team to enable the best level of function possible for the patient and family.

Identification of problems

Assumptions can be dangerous. Each person has individual needs, so each one's aims and expectations will be different. As has been said, needs can be identified as physical, emotional, social and spiritual, and will become apparent through skilled communication with the patient and carer. It can be helpful to clarify with the patient and carer, towards the close of the interview, the areas they see as most important and discuss how best to address these issues.

The progression of MND is unpredictable, and detailed discussion with the patient and carer of what might happen in the future is only helpful if specific issues are of concern to the individual. It can, however, be helpful for the health professional to formulate ideas of possible progression of the illness, to improve planning for the future, particularly where equipment is needed or where future appointments may take some time to plan.

Establish relationships

It is a truism that first impressions are crucial in any situation where two people are hoping to build up a relationship.

(Robbins, 1989).

Establishing a therapeutic relationship with the patient and family takes time and commitment, but first impressions are vital to the process. Trust grows through empathetic listening, and a knowledge of the possible problems and progression of the disease can help the patient to feel more secure.

Having an illness which will shorten a person's life significantly changes that person's concept of self. This in turn affects the hopes and expectations of the entire family. Establishing a relationship with the family based on mutual respect and unconditional positive regard allows them to express their worries and work towards building a new self-image through which they can continue to grow and develop.

Future care planning

Once problems have been identified, it will be necessary to determine those which are most important to the patient and carer. Through this, it will be possible to formulate aims and objectives specific to the individual (see Chapter 3).

Where the initial assessment has been carried out by a consultant, individual members of the multidisciplinary team will be asked to make their assessment. In some cases, there will be little need for intervention at this stage, but once the initial contact has been made, the therapist will be able to make tentative plans for the future. There will be benefit to the patient in that he will know who to contact as the need arises.

Points to remember when planning team treatment:

- detailed assessments of needs of patient and family;
- joint assessments where possible;
- involvement of health professionals before it becomes essential;
- liaison with other teams providing care;
- patient and family as an integral part of the team;
- treatment aims relate to entire team;
- goals may be set by individual team members;
- keyworker holds overview plan and co-ordinates care;
- attention to good communication between team members.

Implementation of care plan

Once plans have been made, it will be necessary to decide how these should be put into action. Time and resources available will have a bearing on this, since the duration of the intervention will last throughout the life of the patient and, for one or more team members, into bereavement in the form of support for the surviving relative(s).

Liaison within the team is vital to avoid duplication of work. The keyworker should help with co-ordination of care input but communication is the responsibility of every member of the team.

Review and reassessment

It is unlikely that this will be a formal process. Use of formal assessment procedures highlight improvement. In treatment of degenerative disease, formal procedures only serve to reinforce deterioration. It will, however, be necessary to monitor the effectiveness of treatment and care being offered and where necessary modification should be considered. This can be achieved by discussion with the patient and carer and is usually an ongoing process.

TYPE OF ASSESSMENT

Establishing the most effective method of assessment of needs merits discussion. MND presents in different forms with the possible progression of the illness varying from a few months to more than five years. Sinaki and Mulder (1978) discuss the advantages of 'classifying patients as to the rapidity of their illness, the site of onset of their disease and the stage of their disability'. Whilst the approach to care will differ between a person with a rapidly progressing disease and one where the progression of the disease is slower, it is not always possible to identify this with any degree of certainty in the initial stages.

Neurological assessments available do not allow for the variety of problems found in people with MND and whilst scored tests may be of use for later research, they are of little functional value where deterioration is expected.

Problem-orientated medical records (POMR) are used in some hospitals. This system can be used by all members of the team to record problems, divided into active (where solutions can be sought) and passive (difficulties worthy of note but over which no action can be taken). It can be argued that this is a negative method of assessment – dwelling on problems (Cantrell in Goodwill and Chamberlain, 1988); other practical drawbacks are that the standard form does not allow for family history or support available from family and friends.

Centrally held records may be of little use to a community team whose members may be working from different bases and whose main form of communication is the telephone. Initial referrals to individual members of the team should be as full as is practical and regular updating by written reporting or verbal communication is vital.

Method of assessment

Assessment can, therefore, be approached as follows:

Framework

Suggested areas of discussion:

- history of illness – first indications, tests, other doctors involved to date;
- occupational history;
- present symptoms/worries;
- current medication;
- home situation;
- family tree;
- personal relationships;
- significant future events for the family;
- main carer(s);
- financial situation;
- physical examination;

- religious beliefs;
- insight of patient and family;
- discussion of priorities of management;
- formulation of action plan with patient and family;
- follow-up appointments.

The initial assessment is usually undertaken by the consultant who intends to continue caring for the patient and family through the course of the illness, and is vital in establishing a relationship between consultant and patient. Information will usually be obtained by:

Direct questioning

Many people are happy to talk about themselves given an interested ear and open questions – for example, what are your main worries at this time? They are less happy to talk about problems which they often see as moans or grumbles.

An open question about an area of possible concern will often be met with a negative answer, whilst a more specific question will elicit information. For example, a patient asked if sleeping was a problem answered 'no', but when asked how long he slept at night revealed that he slept for an hour or two before waking, then could not get back to sleep.

Some people would not identify this as a problem but this patient was then unable to get back to sleep, became uncomfortable lying in bed and had to disturb his wife to turn him. Further questions revealed that he was becoming increasingly concerned that his wife was overtired as a result of the disturbed nights. Following discussion, a pressure-relieving mattress and night sedation were suggested, which relieved the problem.

Observation

Observation of verbal responses and the non-verbal cues behind verbal responses gives insight into true feelings. Where the two are at variance, the non-verbal cue may be closer to the true feeling. This should be noted and, if appropriate, can be explored with the patient and family at the time or later in the interview.

Care should be taken when using observation as a tool to exploration in the early stages of a relationship. An interview can be a stressful situation for many people with the result that they react in a tense manner. As the therapeutic relationship grows, anxiety usually diminishes and observation of non-verbal cues is more reliable.

ASSESSMENT BY MEMBERS OF THE TEAM

Once the medical and psychological assessment has been completed, referral to other members of the multidisciplinary team should be made as necessary. Where possible, joint assessments reduce repetition for the patient and should be encouraged.

MND is comparatively rare and many community health professionals see few, if any, people with the illness. Where diagnosis is made following a hospital admission to the neurological department, it can prove helpful if assessments are made by members of the neurological team at that time. It should then be possible for the hospital team to discuss any problems discovered with the community team on or prior to discharge home.

Areas which may be causing concern are discussed in the following sections.

Mobility

This may be addressed from different angles by different members of the team. The physiotherapist will assess the ability of the patient to move limbs, trunk and neck. Where the patient is still able to walk, walking aids may be provided. Exercises to maintain functional movement for as long as possible and prevent stiffness or physical deformity will be taught.

Transferring the patient from chair, bed or toilet/commode will be assessed by the physiotherapist. Help and advice in this area can be given to the patient and carer as necessary. Methods of helping a person get up from the floor may also be taught since however carefully the patient moves, there will be times when falls occur.

The occupational therapist will assess functional mobility since she has knowledge of equipment which can help to maintain independence for as long as possible. Appendix B lists a number of items and their sources which can be particularly helpful to people with MND.

The progression of the disease is erratic and unpredictable. Better results will be achieved if realistic, attainable short-term goals are set rather than longer-term projects which will need to be altered frequently if they are to be achieved. An example of this may occur if the patient wishes to continue working. It may be necessary to negotiate part-time hours or more work from home, if full-time working causes exhaustion.

Concern with matters of personal care is an area many people take for granted. Loss of mobility can result in difficulties with washing, bathing, use of the toilet, dressing, comfort (sitting in a chair or lying in bed), eating and drinking. Many of these difficulties can at least be improved by use of compensatory movements and equipment. The occupational therapist will assess these areas and, where problems exist, should be able to offer suggestions to help.

Advice on energy-saving techniques may also be necessary and time may need to be spent talking with the patient and carer about accepting help in the home. For many people this is an emotionally charged area, especially if they do not have extended family support, and extra help entails introduction of a stranger into the home. If help is not introduced early in the illness, the patient becomes used to being cared for by one family member, who can be overwhelmed by the ensuing tasks.

If walking becomes difficult, quality of life may be improved by provision of a wheelchair. Suggesting the use of a wheelchair requires sensitivity since its use reinforces deterioration and changes a person's self-image. Society's concept of disability is gradually becoming more positive but there is still a tendency to view a person in a wheelchair as inferior. It may be necessary to make the suggestion and allow time for thought and discussion with the family before the idea is accepted.

Mobility also relates to the ability of the patient to use public or private transport. Consideration of the use of a car with adapted controls to be used by the patient, or alterations to a private car to enable the patient and wheelchair to be transported, falls to the occupational therapist. An assessment at a centre specializing in this area of work may be required to ensure that the most appropriate vehicle is obtained.

The social worker may need to be involved to advise on financial assistance relating to matters of mobility. Benefits may be available to enable or help with purchase of a suitable vehicle. If the patient wishes to continue driving the insurance company should be notified that the patient has MND. This should not affect the insurance premium but will ensure that the insurance cover is still valid in the event of an accident.

Home assessments

In some areas of the country, community physiotherapists are employed to visit and advise people in their own homes. This can be particularly useful if there is difficulty transporting the patient to the physiotherapy department. Where possible, community physiotherapists aim to teach carers to deal with problems that arise, but regular visits may be necessary to monitor developments.

Home assessment by the occupational therapist will be necessary at an early stage. Patients and their families, if given the opportunity, will discuss areas of concern to them. Observation on the part of the occupational therapist will also identify areas of possible future concern.

Many patients are reluctant to look too far into the future and may reject suggestions which would alter their homes, even if they would improve their quality of life. Solutions which result in the least disruption but effect the maximum benefit to the patient are recommended in these situations.

Liaison with social services and the local environmental health department by the occupational therapist will usually be needed to fund major alterations or extensions to property. If major work is contemplated, it needs to be started early if it is to be completed before it becomes essential.

Quality of life can be improved for people with MND by provision of an environmental control system (Possum or Steeper in UK). These allow various elements of the environment, e.g. turning lights on and off, using the telephone or television, to be controlled by using one switch fed through a computer-based control system. The Possum and Steeper systems also allow for communication by word processor and can be linked to a printer. This makes them both suitable systems for use by people with MND.

Assessment is made by a representative of the medical officer of health for the area and an occupational therapist, following referral by the general practitioner, if funding is sought through the health authority. Private funding is possible but costly.

Speech and swallowing

Assessment by the speech and language therapist should be considered even if dysarthria or dysphagia appear to be mild. Impairment to speech or swallowing can be the result of dysfunction in one of many areas and detailed assessment will be necessary to identify the problem.

Exercises can be suggested to maintain maximum function for as long as possible, and conscious attention to normally unconscious acts can help, particularly with swallowing and articulation.

Speech may lose volume if the chest muscles become weak. Breathing exercises may be taught by the physiotherapist or speech and language therapist to maintain maximum strength. In addition to improving the quality of speech, breathing exercises can also help to alleviate anxiety caused by breathlessness.

Nutritional needs

The role of the dietitian may overlap with that of the speech and language therapist over the best consistency of food. Where swallowing problems are present, thought should be given to texture of food. This may be addressed by either the dietitian or the speech and language therapist.

Nutritional needs will be assessed by the dietitian. Techniques for improving the calorific value of food consumed can help to prevent severe weight loss and fatigue caused by insufficient intake of food.

Where dysphagia is severe, parenteral feeding (by nasogastric tube or percutaneous gastrostomy) may need consideration (see Chapter 6). If performed, the dietitian will assess the dietary requirements of the patient and recommend the appropriate nutritional intake.

Social problems and benefits

The benefit system in Great Britain, whilst planned to be user friendly, can be confusing and help may be needed to ensure appropriate claims are made. The social worker will be able to assess and advise on financial help available.

The counselling skills of the social worker will also be required in supporting the patient and family through the course of the illness.

CARE IN THE COMMUNITY

All disabled people would get a good deal if unlimited funding were available for community care. They would have individual assessments of need to identify care packages and equipment required for independent living.

(Swain, 1993).

The 1990 NHS and Community Care Act came into force in the UK on 1 April 1993. It aims to replace potentially fragmented social care from local authorities, and health care from community health services, with a co-ordinated service based on the needs of the patient and the carers. Care needs assessments are sought from the multidisciplinary team by a care manager who, in consultation with the patient and multidisciplinary team, constructs a care package to meet their needs.

Care packages are not new; they have been used in the past to enable people with physical disabilities or learning disabilities to continue to live at home with as much independence as possible. Funding care packages has been difficult in the past, as has accessing the appropriate care. This has led, in many cases, to a fragmented service. Unfortunately the care management budget is not limitless, but it is hoped that by a holistic assessment of care needs and financial organization by one person, a co-ordinated whole will be achieved.

Residential care is another area of concern for care management. It is hoped that by use of care packages, more people will be able to continue to live at home. However, this may not always be possible and residential care may be necessary.

One of the major changes introduced by the 1990 Act is the transfer of funds previously available through the social security system for residential and nursing home places in the private sector to local authorities. Placement of people with limited financial means will henceforth (from 1 April 1993) be at the discretion of social services.

(Browning, 1992).

Continuing care hospital beds have reduced over recent years and the gap that this has created has been filled by an increase in residential and nursing home beds. This can place a person with MND and the family in a dilemma, since residential care is often needed when the patient's condition has deteriorated to a level where a residential home would be unable to offer sufficient care. Many nursing homes find themselves in a similar position.

Nursing home care can cost between £250 and £400 plus per week. Application for financial help towards funding such care has to be made through a care manager who, following financial assessment, may be able to recommend the standard grant and/or additional funds to pay any shortfall. Unfortunately, in many cases, at least some of the cost of nursing home care has to be met by the patient or relatives.

It is hoped that care managers will be in a position to advise on appropriate services available locally, although many areas of the country would appear to have limited provision of suitable resources. Community care has often been regarded as the 'Cinderella' service (Browning) and its transformation may take some time to complete.

SPECIALIST ASSESSMENT CENTRES AND FACILITIES

Services available for people with MND vary depending on the health and social professionals working in a given area. In an attempt to provide appropriate facilities and standardize care, assessment units and pilot care studies have been run in different parts of the country. The following section is a summary of these services.

Mary Marlborough Centre

People with severe disabilities often experience problems that cannot be solved adequately within their locality by local staff. Specialist assessment units aim to provide a specialist service to help people with severe disabilities to live as independently as possible.

Mary Marlborough Centre, at the Nuffield Orthopaedic Hospital in Oxford, has provided a specialist service for over 30 years for people suffering from a number of conditions including MND. They aim to provide a unique problem-solving service which is directed towards the following objectives:

- enhance an individual's quality of life
- maintain people in their own environment
- alleviate and reduce pain
- avoid deformity and maintain function
- reduce strain on carer

- diminish demands on statutory services
- help employees stay at work longer
- maintain morale, dignity and comfort for client/carer.

The centre aims to assess most people in their own homes using an outreach team of therapists working in liaison with the local multidisciplinary team. They work within the Oxford region and their team of specialists includes a consultant in rehabilitation medicine, occupational therapists, physiotherapists, rehabilitation engineers, nurses, a speech and language therapist, a clinical psychologist, horticultural therapist and recreational therapist. The choice of therapist is decided by the presenting problem/s.

Once the problem/s have been identified, recommendations are made which may involve the patient and carer in a short stay at the centre for trying or fitting of equipment.

MNDA centres

Our vision is to provide care that responds to the needs of INDIVIDUALS. We also intend to play a leading role in raising standards of education, training and care co-ordination through building on our links with GP's, social services, voluntary agencies and hospices.

(Leigh, in Thumb Print, *1993).*

The first MNDA centre was opened at the Maudsley Hospital, London, in November 1993. It is hoped that more will be opened in the future, eventually giving any person with MND access to a centre no further than two hours journey time away, in England, Northern Ireland and Wales.

The need for appropriate care is now more widely recognized, but co-ordination of such care is still sadly lacking in many areas of the country. The MNDA centres aim to house therapeutic, clinical and scientific work in one unit which, it is hoped, will focus the skills of the multidisciplinary team to benefit patients, in addition to co-ordinating care.

It is intended that these centres will:

- hold a clinic at regular intervals – not less than one month apart – on a 'drop in' or appointment basis;
- enable the patient to see the same consultant or registrar at each visit;
- enable the patient to have access to a full range of paramedical staff, appropriate to their needs;
- provide specified standards of health care;
- liaise with health professionals in the patient's home area.

The MNDA accept that they would need to continue to grant fund the research projects through the existing system and may also be required to pay for additional clinicians, therapists, co-ordinators or administrators where necessary. Meeting the running costs for the centres, it is hoped, will become a focus for fund-raising efforts. It is thought that the benefits of these centres will provide sufficient impetus to enable adequate funding to be obtained.

Collaborative care planning

The collaborative care plan pilot study was set up at six acute hospitals in the West Midlands in April 1990 and ran for a period of six months. The studies were limited to in-patient care and of the six hospitals taking part, one – Queen Elizabeth Hospital, Birmingham – was concerned with its application to patients with MND.

Collaborative care planning uses a multidisciplinary team approach to assessment, planning implementation and evaluation of care in co-operation with the patient. The aim of employing this approach is to make effective use of resources and ensure that care is clearly defined, planned, implemented, monitored and audited. Importance was placed on definition of the treatment period from pre-admission through to discharge planning and follow-up care in the community.

Whilst setting up and implementing this system required effort, benefits of the pilot study were identified:

- team building for patient and therapists;
- patients having contact telephone numbers for the various therapists involved in their care;
- identification of a keyworker;
- rapid confirmation of diagnosis by organizing pre-planned and booked investigations;
- improved communication between disciplines;
- clearer overview of individual case management.

Neuro-care approach to motor neurone disease

This study, carried out in Romford, Essex, between April 1990 and September 1992, was part of a 'wider strategy of care' which was set up to offer treatment to patients suffering from several other progressive neurological conditions. The study involved 12 unselected patients with MND, i.e. all new MND patients diagnosed by the local neurological team.

The basic features of the strategy for all conditions are: management by a multidisciplinary team, recognition of the need for information and support, special attention to the whole person, and involvement of the patient and relatives in decision making.

(Oxtoby and Eikaas, 1993).

Principles of care included:

- attention to the method by which the diagnosis was given;
- care by a multidisciplinary team;
- use of a co-ordinator/counsellor;
- continuing care from diagnosis to death and bereavement follow-up;
- location of care encompassed time in hospital and care at home.

Generally it was thought that there were disadvantages to addressing several conditions within the same study, but benefits of this type of care included:

- co-ordinated care planning and implementation;
- support for patient and carers available when needed;
- improved quality of life for patient and carer;
- support for health professionals working within the team.

Both multidisciplinary pilot studies reported improvement of care for the patient and carers. Despite the pain that accompanies working with people suffering from a severely disabling neurological illness, working as part of a team provides support and enables the team members to deliver good quality care.

CONCLUSION

Detailed assessment is essential if the needs of the patient and family are to be met. Whilst it may seem an arduous task, careful planning for intervention is more effective for the patient and less stressful for the health professional in the long term.

Involvement of health professionals at an early stage maximizes use of resources by enabling planning and reducing the need for crisis intervention.

Introduction of the Government paper on *Care in the Community* has underlined the need for assessment and, whilst there would appear to be discrepancy between the needs of the patient and resources available in many areas, there is hope that in future this will be reduced to provide a good, standard level of care for all patients, regardless of their location.

REFERENCES

Browning, D. (1992) Getting ready for change. *B.M.J.*, **305**, 1415–18.
Goodwill, C.J. and Chamberlain, M.A. (eds) (1988) *Rehabilitation of the Physically Disabled Adult*, Chapman & Hall, London.

Kaye, P. (1991) *Symptom Control in Hospice and Palliative Care* (3rd edn), Hospice Education Institute, Connecticut, USA.

Newrick, P. G. and Langton-Hewer, R. (1984) MND: can we do better? *B.M.J.*, **289**, 539–42.

Oxtoby, M. and Eikaas, M. (1993) Multidisciplinary management from day one: the neuro-care approach to motor neurone disease. *Palliative Medicine*, **7** (suppl. 2), 31–6.

Robbins, J. (1989) *Caring For The Dying Patient And The Family* (2nd edn), Harper and Row, London.

Sinaki, M. and Mulder, D. (1978) Rehabilitation techniques for patients with amyotrophic lateral sclerosis. *Mayo. Clin. Proc.*, **53**, 173–8.

Swain, P. (1993) Helping disabled people – the user's view. *B.M.J.*, **306**, 990–2.

Thumb Print (1993) Winter edition, the magazine of the Motor Neurone Disease Association, Northampton, England.

Turner, A., Foster, M. and Johnson, S. (eds) (1992) *Occupational Therapy and Physical Dysfunction*, Churchill Livingstone, Edinburgh.

FURTHER READING

Ainsworth-Smith, A. and Speck, P. (1982) *Letting Go*, SPCK, London.

Cardy, P. (1992) *MNDA Centres*, MNDA, PO Box 246, Northampton.

Cochrane, G. (1987) *The Management of Motor Neurone Disease*, Churchill Livingstone, Edinburgh.

Gross, R. (1992) *Psychology* (2nd edn), Hodder and Stoughton, London.

Mearns, D. and Thorne, B. (1992) *Person Centred Counselling in Action*, Sage Publications, London.

PART THREE

Practical Considerations

> I wish with all my heart and soul that I had not written this paper; for then I should still be where I spent five years' training to be, and where I planned to spend these years of my life, at work as a civil engineer, looking forward to coming home and playing football with my son. It would also mean, of course, that I would not have had to endure this agonising and devastating illness, motor neurone disease.
>
> *(Carus, 1980).*

These words form the introduction to a paper by Roger Carus, published in the *British Medical Journal* just after his death from motor neurone disease in 1979. The paper following that introduction is a chronicle of ineptitude and missed opportunities on the part of many of the people involved in his care, and the anger, frustration and isolation that Mr Carus felt, being faced with this incurable illness.

Theoretical frameworks form the foundation to practice and help to order thinking. This book so far has been concerned with mainly theoretical issues. This section aims to show how theory can be put into practice – how use of a multidisciplinary team approach, patient-centred assessment, treatment planning, intervention and evaluation can support both patient and carer through the various stages of this illness.

> ... the illness is physical but given adequate help it is not too difficult to cope with. It is the emotional and mental stresses which are more of a problem.
>
> *(Holden, 1980).*

This section will also attempt to convey the thoughts and feelings of people living with this illness and those who care for them, about issues that they find important. Patients and their families are often good teachers and, where health professionals are prepared to learn from them, it is possible to formulate and improve the care they can offer.

The chapters in this section relate to the four identifiable stages of the progression of the illness. The clinical features addressed in each chapter will often be present at other stages of the disease; the stage at which they are discussed is the stage at which they are usually most troublesome to the patient.

Primary care | 5

I was devastated ... We worked it out, what it was –
or what we thought it was. Celia, my wife, and I – we
sat and we discussed it, and we knew what was coming
really. But you can never prepare yourself for when
somebody actually tells you. You might know it within
yourself but when somebody tells you you've got it,
(MND), that's when it's a different ball-game.
  (Barry Stevenson-Cleaver, 1989, in Foreman, 1991).

INTRODUCTION

Barry knew, before diagnosis, that there was a possibility he had motor
neurone disease. He had worked in the army medical corps and, since he
followed a strict fitness programme, he knew by his performance levels
that he was becoming weaker. Many people have not heard of MND
before and if they have, it may be just a name. They are unprepared for
what is to come.

The initial symptoms of MND are usually minor. Weakness in a hand
or arm, tripping over for no reason, generally increased clumsiness or
slurring of speech. It is unlikely that a family doctor will think of MND
as the first choice of diagnosis and people with the illness may be referred
to two or three different consultants before arriving at the neurologist for
tests.

DIAGNOSIS

A diagnosis of MND is established following neurological tests and clinical
examination. In some cases it may be obvious, in others more obscure.
Once the diagnosis is confirmed, the neurologist may be faced with a
dilemma – whether the patient should be informed of their diagnosis.

Until comparatively recently, the role of the consultant was perceived to be somewhere between autocracy and paternalism. Over the past few years, the relationship between consultant and patient has changed. In some cases, it has developed into a partnership where information passes naturally between the people concerned. Unfortunately this is not always the case and, where it is not, the medical practitioner may be concerned as to whether the patient should be informed of their diagnosis.

The effects of motor neurone disease are such that they cannot be ignored for long. If a person is not told, fear and anxiety develop. Most people with the disease have found the effects most frightening, before the diagnosis was confirmed. However devastating it may be to know the diagnosis, uncertainty is worse.

Most health professionals working with people suffering from a terminal illness find that they need to address the issue of **how** to share the information rather than **whether** to share the information with their clients or patients. It has been found that the way in which bad news is imparted has a significant bearing on the individual's future ability to cope with their illness (Fallowfield, 1993).

BREAKING BAD NEWS

Communicating bad news is a skill that has, until recently, been generally neglected by medical schools. Whilst more time is now allocated to communication skills for medical practitioners, it would appear to be insufficient since many doctors still feel ill-prepared to handle situations in which they have to impart difficult information.

Most health professionals have need to impart bad news at some time in their careers. This may not involve communication of a serious diagnosis, but any information that results in change for the patient needs to be addressed with care and sensitivity.

The task should never be easy. The information given will significantly alter the lives of the patients and the people around them. The major consideration for the health professional is that they are not responsible for the situation that has happened, but they are responsible for putting the information across in the kindest and most appropriate way possible.

The aims are positive. Sharing information, whether good or bad, forms the basis of trust on which relationships can be built. It is an exchange of information and, even if this information is not good, it serves to reduce uncertainty. The way in which the diagnosis can be imparted in a positive, constructive manner is illustrated in the following case study.

George, a single gentleman in his mid-forties, was referred to the neurologist by his general practitioner for assessment as a result of progressive weakness and loss of balance. He was admitted to hospital for five days to undergo tests. At the end of this time a positive diagnosis of MND was reached.

The test results were received on a Friday afternoon. George was due to be discharged from hospital that day, but it was thought by the neurological team to be unsatisfactory to inform him of his diagnosis, on his own, and then send him home to face the weekend alone with the news.

Once the news had been broken, he was offered the opportunity to stay in over the weekend until Tuesday or Wednesday, to allow time for him to assimilate the information, ask questions and meet the hospital team of therapists who could assess his initial needs.

When George returned home, he had some idea of how he might face the future. The hospital therapists contacted the community therapists in George's home town and his treatment continued with trips back to see the neurologist for review appointments.

Principles of breaking bad news are summarized in the following sections.

Preparation

Consultations with this patient group should be planned in advance. Privacy is essential. It may not always be easy to provide a separate room for this purpose in the ward setting, but it is necessary. Curtains and screens create an illusion of seclusion, but voices can be overheard and misunderstandings can result.

Adequate time should be allowed not only for the consultation but also to check details beforehand. It is very easy to rush difficult meetings on the pretext of having little time. If considered honestly, this will usually be found to be rooted in the anxiety of the health professional. The manner in which the interview is conducted reflects the doctor's willingness to give time.

Attention to detail helps to convey empathy. This includes ensuring that there will be no interruptions and arranging for a colleague to deal with pagers or emergency calls.

Joint interviews can have many benefits. Asking that the patient bring a relative or friend to an out-patient appointment, or arranging the interview during visiting time if this ensures the presence of a significant person on the ward, reduces the patient's feelings of vulnerability, and communicates sensitivity on the part of the health professional.

Involvement of another member of the healthcare team can also be beneficial. The presence of two members of the team can share the load and provides an alternative point of reference for the patient after the interview has ended.

Use of questions

How the interview is conducted will depend to a great extent on the individual health professional. It will be necessary to understand how much information has been assimilated by the patient and family to date before moving forward. Questioning will give an idea as to how much change will be necessary in the patient's thinking. If the patient has already progressed towards the thought that the condition may be serious, the movement will be less than for the patient who believes he is suffering from a trapped nerve which could be corrected by time or surgery.

Asking questions will also be helpful in finding out the amount of information the patient wants to hear. Many people have not heard of MND or, if they have, their knowledge may be sketchy. It has been found that giving too much information too soon can lead to confusion, as the patient tries to make sense of all the information he is being given.

Framework

Use of a framework can help in the retention of information. For example, informing someone that you are 'about to give them two pieces of information: firstly . . .', can help to structure that person's thinking, enabling assimilation of the facts.

Language

Health professionals often use a language of their own which should be confined to use with other health professionals. In this context, the language used should be simple and unambiguous, and should avoid the use of jargon and euphemisms. People in this situation have difficulty remembering information; simplicity aids memory.

Words are powerful tools, their impact can be far reaching. Careful listening to patients can give clues to the words that are significant in their lives. This can be particularly important when discussing emotions – where, for instance, there is a difference between sadness and depression, or anger and irritation.

Repetition

People often perceive what is said in different ways. By acknowledging this with the patient, and asking him to repeat what he understands of what has been said to him, misconceptions can be kept to a minimum.

Provision of information

A diagnosis of MND may have little meaning to many people who find they are developing the illness. It has been found that 'a "gradual dawning" is probably better than "brutal telling" ' (Langton-Hewer, in Goodwill and Chamberlain, 1988), since any treatment available is symptomatic.

The use of diagrams and leaflets to reinforce information should be considered. Leaflets produced by the MNDA can be sent on request to health professionals and people with MND and their families.

The progression of the disease is so variable that to inform the patient of problems, many of which will not be relevant to him, would be confusing and unnecessary. Giving basic information about what is happening in the present is usually sufficient and allows for discussion to develop.

It has been found helpful to reinforce areas not affected by the disease. Whilst this would not presume to be a consolation, sight, hearing, incontinence and mental impairment can be a great concern to patients, and reassurance that these areas will not be affected is often beneficial.

The attitude and non-verbal cues of the health professional are vital. The most important piece of information that the patient needs to hear at this stage, is that he is assured of the continued help and support of the healthcare team and that he will not be abandoned and left to fight on alone. The patient needs verbal reassurance of this, but the empathetic understanding and actions of the health professionals involved in his care convey much of this message.

Assurance of continued support opens the door to future conversations and enables the patient and family to return or contact people in the team to ask questions. These questions should be answered honestly but with sensitivity. Care should be taken to listen to the question and to answer what is asked. In this way, the patient remains in control of the information he receives and feels he can ask further questions up to the level at which he can cope.

An early follow-up appointment and the provision of points of contact in the patient's area can be particularly helpful. The MNDA, in addition to publishing leaflets, runs a helpline between 9 a.m. and 10 p.m. each weekday, providing a useful point of contact.

FACING LIFE-THREATENING ILLNESS

Few people in our society are encouraged to think about the end of their life. Death and dying are generally viewed as taboo subjects, best put off until later. The way in which people adjust to a diagnosis of MND will depend to a large extent on their previous thoughts in relation to this subject and their personality, since they will react in character.

The will to live is a strong basic human instinct and any threat to it can be devastating. Whilst most people are aware academically that they will not live for ever, facing the probability that their life will end sooner rather than later requires a major alteration of thought.

Thought processes are accompanied by a variety of differing emotions, and feelings can be confusing both to the patient and family. It is possible to experience different emotions at the same time, just as it is possible to shift through different emotional states in a short space of time.

Emotions in this situation have been likened to the tide. They wash over a person in an intense manner for a time, and then recede. Studies have been made into the ways in which people react on being told they have an incurable illness. Perhaps the best known work in this area was led by Elisabeth Kubler-Ross (1970) who found that people passed through various stages on the way to recovering their equilibrium in the face of terminal illness. These emotions are summarized in the following sections.

Shock and denial

Shock has the effect of numbing the mind. When people are given bad news, they often have difficulty in remembering what has been said. 'This can't be happening to me' is often an early reaction. There is a positive aspect to shock: it introduces a layer of insulation between the person and reality, which enables the full effect of the news to sink in gradually.

Denial is characterized by phrases such as 'I will not believe that this is happening to me.' It often causes a search for a different diagnosis of a less severe kind, and usually passes after the initial shock subsides.

Denial is a common defence mechanism – the inability to acknowledge the seriousness of the situation as it relates to the individual. Through the progression of the illness, the patient will usually experience periods when he acknowledges the reality of the situation interspersed with periods of denial or partial denial. This can help the patient to live with the possibility of death and an uncertain future.

Continuous denial can be destructive if it persists, since it may block attempts by others to provide help as the disease progresses and the person becomes weaker. If this occurs, skilled psychological help may be necessary to challenge the denial and enable the person to move forward. However, in most cases denial, if present, serves to protect the person as he works through the pertinent issues surrounding the diagnosis.

Isolation

MND, as has been stated, is still a condition of which most people have little understanding or knowledge. The reaction of many people to their diagnosis has been 'At least it's not cancer or multiple sclerosis', both of which are better known.

Feelings of isolation are usually caused by people, both professionals and others, who have little experience of MND and are unaware of the needs of this patient group. Searching for information can be frustrating and adds to the isolation. Introduction to the MNDA or health professionals who have experience in this area of work can help to reduce feelings of isolation.

Anger

Anger usually emerges when the effects of shock and denial begin to lessen. It is easy to understand why a person might react angrily in having to adjust to a life-threatening illness. It is not so easy to cope with the effects of anger and the form it may take.

Anger may be displaced from its original target and characterized by statements such as: 'The doctor who made the diagnosis should have known earlier'; 'Everyone else in the world seems to be well and happy'; 'How can anyone believe in a God when people still contract incurable illnesses?' It may be directed at the person closest to the patient who is trying to help, an occurrence which may seem perverse, but anger can be difficult to express outside a secure relationship.

Conversely, it can happen that because a person has a life-threatening illness, unacceptable angry behaviour may be allowed to continue unchallenged. This results in resentment building within the relationship, whether it be between the patient and their relatives or health professionals. Acknowledging and exploring the anger rather than ignoring it is less damaging to relationships.

A patient-centred approach to care and the assurance of unconditional positive regard (Rogers) can be constructive in handling anger. Allowing a person the space to express their anger without reacting to it personally can help patients to feel their anger, and direct it more appropriately (see Chapter 6).

Guilt

Responsibility and guilt are inextricably linked. People, in general, are conditioned to fulfil expectations and can therefore feel responsible if they fail. When considered, expectations can often be identified as the hopes of another person and are not always realistic for the individual concerned.

The patient and family may need help to work through these expectations and to establish which of them are realistic and which are not. Encouraging a person's awareness and acceptance of self can help to reduce the negative effects of guilt.

Research has, as yet, been unsuccessful in establishing the cause of MND; however, it is not uncommon for patients to have strong feelings of responsibility for their illness. They may feel there is a possibility that their lifestyle, environment, occupation or some action from the past could have caused the disease. The individual may also feel guilty for the circumstances in which he has to leave his family, or he may feel responsible for wrecking family life. Time should be set aside for discussion and exploration of these issues and, where possible, reassurance or help may be offered.

Guilt can be destructive and if ignored may cause great unhappiness for both the patient and family. It does, however, demonstrate a sensitivity in the individual. 'Guilt may not have a **purpose** as such, but it certainly does signal some positive qualities in the sufferer' (Buckman, 1988). Without this sensitivity, there would be a lack of feeling for others on the part of the individual.

Fear

There are many causes of fear. At the time of diagnosis, the most common fear is of the inability to cope with the prospect of reduced mobility and ability and the issues that this will engender.

Fears may be bound up with losses. Loss of work, status, role within the family or finances. It may equally be concerned with the patient or carer's ability or desire to cope with the new situation. The future may seem much more uncertain. Fear in the face of uncertainty is common and repeated reassurance of continued support by health professionals can reinforce stability and help the patient to cope with this fear.

Whilst many patients may move their thoughts towards acknowledging that life expectancy will be shortened, many people at this stage do not address the fear of death. There is much to be done to enhance and encourage enjoyment of life and time is usually spent working to these ends. Fear of death is usually addressed gradually during the course of the illness and, as such, will be discussed later in this book.

No two people will have the same fears; something that will be frightening to one person may not occur to another. Many people feel guilty if they are afraid, and may be reluctant to show their fear. It will be necessary for the health professional to demonstrate a willingness to share these fears and work with the patient and family to resolve them where possible.

Bargaining

Like denial, bargaining is a defence that may be used in an attempt to postpone the inevitable. It often takes the form of trying to secure a pact with God and may only be alluded to in conversation, if acknowledged at all. At its most basic, it may be expressed as a plea to God through the sentiment 'If I behave myself and go to church each week, will you let me live?'.

It may, however, take a more factual form: 'My son will be coming home from abroad in three weeks. If I can live to see him, I will not ask for anything else'. In this situation, if the deadline is reached, a new bargain is often established.

Bargaining can be seen as an extension of hope, which is necessary for anyone if they are to continue to maintain some quality of life.

Depression and despair

If care is taken to communicate the nature of the diagnosis with sensitivity, depression rarely causes a serious problem at this time. If, however, all hope is destroyed, despair and depression can proliferate.

Reinforcing a person's worth and usefulness and illustrating a willingness to stay with him, even through his most difficult times, can help to preserve hope and thus dispel despair. Encouraging involvement in planning for the present and future can also help to lift a person's mood.

Sadness is a natural reaction to serious illness and an uncertain future and should be distinguished from despair and depression. Despair grows through lack of hope. Depression, characterized by poor sleep patterns, loss of appetite and expression, general exhaustion and tearfulness, may be a reaction to the illness.

Depression is recognized as an integral part of facing terminal illness (Kubler-Ross, 1970) and is associated with the acceptance of a serious illness. It is usually present at some time during the course of this disease. Depression may also be associated with losses. At the time of diagnosis, the patient will be adjusting to his probable loss of future and will experience powerful emotions through this adjustment. These emotions will be experienced repeatedly as the disease progresses as they are related to grieving for the loss of different abilities.

Acceptance and resolution

This, the final stage of facing terminal illness, is reached – if at all – following thought and consideration of the previous issues. As with the other stages, it is rarely final. The usual experience is of a stage through which the patient passes and re-enters from different directions.

Living with MND involves looking at separate issues and losses associated with the illness as they arise. As a new stage of the illness is reached, the process is repeated. It is to be hoped that each loss experienced by the patient with MND can be resolved before the onset of the next.

An illustration of this point is taken from an article by a patient at St Christopher's Hospice, London, when he writes:

'Coming to terms with your illness' is a phrase much used and I wonder what people think the process is. Do they believe that at some point you say to yourself, 'Look, you are in a pickle, but just pull yourself together, make the best of a bad job and, apart from the odd lapse you will be alright'. It is not like that. It is a day-to-day effort to adjust and adapt to a declining capability.

(Holden, 1980).

PRESERVATION OF HOPE

In the depth of your hopes and desires lies your silent knowledge of the beyond;
  And like seeds dreaming beneath the snow your heart dreams of spring.

(Gibran, 1991).

Daily life is made possible by the existence of hope. Everyone has hopes for the future, however long or short the future may be perceived. People with MND and their families are no exception. Hope falls into two categories: false and realistic.

False hope

False hope can be damaging. It can raise expectations for a short while but the pain felt when these expectations are not realized can be severe. False hope is usually offered when a person, health professional or other, is asked a question they feel unable to answer truthfully.

People with MND often fear the loss of ability which accompanies the illness. To this end they may ask such questions as 'Will I lose the power of speech?'. It can be tempting to answer 'No, of course not'. The reality is that no one has any way of knowing until the situation occurs. To give the above as an answer serves to escalate anxiety which, in itself, can cause pain to the patient.

Realistic hope

Realistic hope enables a person to face the future, however uncertain, in the knowledge that he will not be alone. It gives purpose to life and prompts the answer to the question above, 'I do not know if you will lose your speech but if it looks as if you will, we will explore different equipment to help you to communicate'. The following case study underlines this point.

Bill, a 61–year-old gentleman with MND, relied heavily on his electric wheelchair for mobility. As the muscles in his arms became weaker, he began to worry that he would no longer be able to operate the controls on his chair.

This worry became so strong that he asked the junior ward doctor whether his arms would become so weak that he would no longer be able to use his chair. The doctor answered that his arms would never become that weak.

Bill was obviously pleased with the answer, but continued to ask the same question of others. He subsequently asked the occupational therapist who replied that she had no way of knowing if this would happen but if it did appear to be becoming a problem, they would look together into different ways of controlling the chair.

Bill then admitted that his possible loss of mobility was one of his strongest fears. By acknowledging this with him and reassuring him of continued support and involvement, hope for the future was kept alive.

Hope reinforces self-esteem and helps to free individuals to be themselves. As ability decreases a person's self-worth can diminish also. There can be many months or years of life after diagnosis which should be used to the full, not wasted. Life is precious even to a person who, to an outsider, may look to be suffering unendurable disability. Empathy on the part of the carers prevents assumptions being made on the patient's behalf.

'No one knows enough to make a pronouncement of doom upon another human being' (Norman Cousins in Kaye, 1991). Research is being carried out into the effects and possible causes of MND, and it is not unknown for people to live for many years with the disease. Hope allows for positive use to be made of the time available.

NEEDS OF THE PATIENT AND CARER AT THE TIME OF DIAGNOSIS

Individual needs will vary not only from person to person but within the same person at different times. The following summary provides a starting point for areas which may be causing concern to a person at diagnosis of MND and immediately after they have been diagnosed, and the approach needed to address these issues.

Empathetic understanding

Empathy is the ability to see a situation from another person's viewpoint, to 'walk in another person's moccasins' (Brearley and Birchley, 1986). It is the ability to enter another person's world and look at situations as that person sees them. It involves maintaining a grasp on reality whilst being able to move around within another's world.

Most people who have been diagnosed as having MND experience a variety of emotions which can change within a short space of time. At this stage, the patient is often trying to alter his perception of his present and future life, whilst his family, reacting to the same situation, obviously experience emotional responses of their own.

Health professionals involved during this time are in a privileged position. It is at this point that basic relationships are formed. Creating a non-judgemental atmosphere where these emotions can be explored without fear of rejection can help the family to work together and mobilize their own resources to enable them to move forward.

Good communication between the patient and family should be encouraged but, in addition, there may be a need for the patient and/or carer to talk with someone outside the family circle. At times, feelings are experienced that would be difficult to discuss with close family members, since they would be too painful or feel too dangerous to share with someone closely involved. Health professionals can help by providing an opportunity for discussion of these feelings.

Provision of information

There is still much to be learned about the disease process and causes of MND; however, it is possible to obtain information through neurology departments, directly from the MNDA and from some of the health professionals working with this patient group.

People who have been newly diagnosed as having MND should be told of the existence of information sources and encouraged to ask for the information they require.

Consideration of children

In the midst of a new and possibly frightening situation, it can be easy to push children into the background. Some people feel that children are too young to understand about death and dying and should be protected from unpleasant and painful situations. If honest, this usually stems from a fear within the adult of communicating with a child about such matters, and possibly it is an area within the adult that is unresolved.

In the same manner as adults deal with grief and loss in their own way, as it is with children. There is, however, increasing evidence that involving children during the illness and dying progress of a close family member reduces psychological problems later on (Kaye, 1991).

Communication with children is important from the start and, as with adults, a 'gradual dawning' is preferable to bald statements of reality. In many situations, parents are the most appropriate people to talk with their children but may need support and affirmation in order to carry out the task.

Talking with younger children requires a different approach to talking with adults. Children are more visual and use of drawings and stories can be helpful. Situations need to be related to those within the child's understanding and in language with which he or she is familiar. Children need praise particularly when they have been helpful or contributed in some way.

Children may need to be encouraged to ask questions and will only ask what they need to know at that time. Answering the question honestly, but with sensitivity, will allow them to ask for more information in the knowledge that they will not be told about things with which they cannot cope at the time.

Older children and teenagers may find it helpful to talk with a member of the healthcare team. They may be experiencing feelings that are difficult to understand and may feel uncomfortable about burdening their parents or may want to ask questions of their own. Many teenagers prefer to talk to people other than their parents on different issues and this should not be viewed as a rejection.

Many people are aware that a small group of people with MND (between 5–10%) have an inherited form of the illness. This may worry parents or children but, in general, neurologists are happy to discuss such worries with the people concerned. In most cases, people with the familial type of the illness are asked at the time of diagnosis whether they know of any other members within their family who have died as a result of MND or other unexplained paralysing illness. In this way, familial links are usually established at the time of diagnosis.

Caring for a heavily dependent husband or wife can take up much time and emotional energy. Where children are involved within the family unit as a small part of the caring team, they are less likely to feel pushed out and disregarded. In the longer term, they feel that they have been able to make a positive contribution throughout the illness (see also Chapter 8).

Assessment of needs

People who are diagnosed as having an incurable illness often feel that they have failed in some way and their self-esteem becomes very low.

Allowing time for a detailed assessment of their needs shows a serious intent to try and improve life for the patient and family (see Chapter 4).

Early involvement by the multidisciplinary team

Many people diagnosed as having MND are told that the illness is incurable and there is nothing that can be done. This is often taken literally to mean that there is no cure and that any unpleasant symptoms have to be endured, since there is no treatment available. It is important during the initial stage of the illness to ensure that the patient and family are aware of help that can be offered by members of the multidisciplinary team.

If team members are introduced early, a point of contact can be established. Many people find it reassuring to know that help is available should it be needed.

Assurance of continued support

Life suddenly becomes very precarious following the diagnosis of MND. Loneliness and isolation are often the response to feeling that no one cares or can do anything to help. A positive attitude to management and the reassurance that everything possible will be done to enable the patient and family to live life to the full provides hope for the future.

CLINICAL FEATURES

At the time of diagnosis, symptoms are usually mild but knowledge of the possible problems can be helpful when planning patient care.

Weakness

This is due to the progressive degeneration of the motor nerves to muscles in the body. It can also be the result of muscle wasting. Abnormal tiredness may also be experienced and whilst exercise is necessary to maintain mobility, it should not be excessive or for prolonged periods since muscles damaged in this way are unable to regenerate.

Tiredness usually becomes more marked towards the end of the day and can be helped by regular rests taken during the day. Essential tasks should be undertaken in the morning rather than left until later in the day, when it is possible that the person may not feel like expending energy.

Thought should be given to the priority of activities undertaken to maximize energy. Many people wish to be independent in personal care but, if after getting dressed energy levels are exhausted, the person may then be unable to do anything else for the rest of the day.

Pain

The sensory nerves are not affected by MND but it is often thought that people with this illness do not experience pain. In their 1981 study, Saunders, Walsh and Smith found that 40% of their sample of people with MND suffered some pain during their illness. This may be a result of any of four problem areas.

1. Joint stiffness

When movement becomes restricted as a result of weakening muscles, joint stiffness may be experienced. Careful positioning and physiotherapy can help, as can the use of non-steroidal anti-inflammatory medication, which may be administered orally or rectally.

As the disease progresses, joints may lose stability as the muscles weaken. Care should be taken with patient handling and transferring if damage to the joints is to be avoided. EU regulations recently introduced require risk assessments to be performed on all patients who need manual handling by professional care staff. The regulations recommend that lifting of patients should be discouraged and that hoists be used wherever possible.

2. Muscle spasms and cramps

Excess spasticity of the muscles can cause severe pain and disability. The use of anti-spasmodic medication such as baclofen or dantrolene can be helpful. Diazepam can help to relieve spasms but may also exacerbate tiredness.

Spasm in moderation (not to the level of being painful) can help when positioning and transferring people who have limited mobility. This should be taken into account when prescribing anti-spasmodic medication. Over-medication can result in falls if the patient is still able to stand or walk.

Cramps are often one of the first signs that there is a problem in the muscles. They often occur at night, particularly in the legs, and can be helped by diazepam or quinine at night.

3. Skin pressure

Decreasing mobility reduces a person's ability to change positions and, particularly if there is extensive muscle wasting, pressure areas may become red and sore. Use of pressure-relieving cushions and mattresses can help to keep the skin intact and improve patient comfort. It should, however, be noted that use of a pressure-relieving mattress may reduce the mobility of the patient in bed, and so is often contraindicated unless mobility in bed is minimal.

4. Decreasing mobility

Many people present initially with problems of mobility. This is often due to weakening muscles causing foot drop or other difficulties with walking. In some cases, the weakness may be so severe that the patient has begun to experience falls. Physiotherapy exercises can help to delay the effects of muscle weakness but cannot build up muscle strength. This should be explained at the start of treatment to prevent hopes being raised unrealistically.

Where equipment is needed to aid mobility, it should be introduced before its use is essential, but not so early that the patient is unable to see a point to its use. Many people are reluctant to accept equipment until symptoms are uncomfortable or severe. Some patients would rather cope with the unpleasant symptoms than accept equipment at all. Whilst every effort should be made to find an acceptable solution, this may not always be possible. This situation can be difficult for some health professionals to accept but may be a method used by the patient to establish control over his life (see also Chapter 4).

PLANNING FOR THE FUTURE

Once the diagnosis has been confirmed, the patient and family will require time to think through the various implications. For some people it will be a time when they are drawn together as a family to plan for the future. Others may feel lonely and isolated and may need outside help to look forward.

Plans made at this time need to be flexible and may need to be revised. It is a time when the patient and family need to be aware of help that can be offered and the people from whom it can be sought. They also need to be in possession of as much information as they feel necessary in order to plan for the future.

CONCLUSION

It is usually recognized that the time of diagnosis can be difficult for the person with MND and the family. However, it is often not recognized that it can also be a difficult time for the health professional.

Understanding the principles of breaking bad news and the emotions which may be relevant to the patient and family at this time can facilitate greater effectiveness of the health professionals involved in their care. Discussion of possible needs and problems facing these families can reduce feelings of helplessness in the health professional and ensure good quality care for the patient and family.

REFERENCES

Brearley, G. and Birchley, P. (1986) *Introducing Counselling Skills and Techniques*, Faber and Faber, London.

Buckman, R. (1988) *I Don't Know What to Say*, Papermac, Basingstoke.

Carus, R. (1980) Motor neurone disease – a demeaning illness. *B.M.J.*, June 16, 455–6.

Fallowfield, L. (1993) Giving sad and bad news. *The Lancet*, **341**, February 20, 476–8

Foreman, R. (ed.) (1991) *The Time of Our Lives – Reminiscences From Cynthia Spencer House*, Cynthia Spencer House, Manfield Campus, Kettering Rd, Northampton NN3 1AD.

Gibran, K. (1991) *The Prophet*, Pan Books, London.

Goodwill, C. J. and Chamberlain, M. A. (eds) (1988) *Rehabilitation of the Physically Disabled Adult*, Chapman & Hall, London.

Holden, T. (1980) Patiently speaking. *Nursing Times*, June 12, 1035–6.

Kaye, P. (1991) *Symptom Control in Hospice and Palliative Care* (revised edn), Hospice Education Institution, Connecticut, USA.

Kubler-Ross, E. (1970) *On Death and Dying*, Tavistock Publications, London.

Saunders, C., Walsh, T. D. and Smith, M. (1981) in *Hospice – The Living Idea*, (eds C. Saunders, D. H. Summers and N. Teller), Edward Arnold, London, p. 121.

FURTHER READING

Brewin, T. (1991) Three ways of giving bad news. *The Lancet*, **337**, May 18, 1207–9.

Buckman, R. (1984) Breaking bad news: why is it still so difficult? *B.M.J.*, **288**, May 26, 1597–90.

Finlay, I. and Dallimore, D. (1991) Your child is dead. *B.M.J.*, **302**, June 22, 1524–5.

Lamerton, R. (1985) *Care of the Dying* (revised edn), Penguin Books, Harmondsworth, England.

McLauchlan, C.A.J. (1990) Handling distressed relatives and breaking bad news. *B.M.J.*, **301**, November 17, 1145–9.

Stedeford, A. (1984) *Facing Death (Patients, Families and Professionals)*, Heinemann, Medical Books, London.

Wooley, H., Stein, A., Forrest, G. C. and Baum, J. D. (1989) Imparting the diagnosis of life threatening illness in children. *B.M.J.*, **298**, June 17, 1623–6.

6

Continuing care

There is a world of difference between looking after a person's needs and caring for them.

(Paul Whiting, 1992).

INTRODUCTION

Paul was 38 years old when he was diagnosed as having motor neurone disease. He was a fiercely independent young man who, at the time of his diagnosis, was unmarried, worked hard and lived with his brother. The words at the beginning of this chapter were given as the response to being asked what he thought was the most important aspect of providing care for people in his position.

These were heartfelt words. In the time between diagnosis and when they were spoken (about 18 months), he had had a succession of carers in his home because of his declining capabilities. Many of them were prepared to look after his physical needs, but became exasperated by what they saw as continual demands. Paul had always demanded high standards of himself and felt unwilling to compromise these as a result of his illness.

Few of the carers were prepared to try to understand why Paul felt the way he did, and how the illness was affecting him as a whole person. They saw their job as looking after his physical needs rather than caring for him. For the few who did try to understand, life was challenging but the benefits achieved through a caring relationship were well worth the effort.

The time between diagnosis and terminal care, termed here as continuing care, involves living daily with an ever-decreasing capability. For the patient, this means waking up each morning feeling well, often forgetting that some of his muscles are paralysed, until he tries to move or get out of bed. For the main carer, it often means walking a tightrope of emotions, offering help where the patient is no longer able to perform tasks independently but being aware that this help may be rejected. As time passes, the carer often feels that she is living life for two people.

For other family members it can mean more tasks to be done about the house to help share the load. A child may be required to help one of the parents in areas of personal care, but in return receives much less attention from either parent.

The period between diagnosis and terminal care can span many months or years and change rarely occurs overnight. At the time of diagnosis, the patient may require very little help and life continues much the same as before. Whilst this stage presents many problems and painful emotions, the human mind is resilient and with time and help, efforts usually return to focus on living and achieving once more.

As the effects of the illness become apparent, the family usually adapt by increasing their input of care to meet the need. Unfortunately, however, there usually comes a time when the carer is giving as much as she is able, but this still does not seem to be enough. If this stage is reached without help from outside agencies, it can be a crisis point for the carer since she is required to admit failure within herself.

Where the multidisciplinary team have been involved from the early stage of the illness, they can usually recognize the pressures that begin to build up and can intervene to avert a crisis. In some cases, however, it may require a crisis within the family to precipitate change and, again, where the team have been involved early, they are familiar with the family and their needs and are better placed to help them find a resolution. Planned management of care for people with degenerative illnesses such as MND should enable the healthcare team to become gradually involved through the continuing care of the patient and family, and place the team members in a position to offer help as and when it is needed.

INTERVENTION

Application of Maslow's hierarchy of needs forms a framework around which issues that are important to many people at this stage of the illness can be considered. Humanistic theories recognize the individual's ability to develop potential through a healthy self-concept, referred to in this setting as self-actualization. Since Maslow recognized that motivation to develop towards self-actualization required that basic needs be fulfilled before needs further up the scale could be addressed, this chapter will address issues similarly.

PHYSIOLOGICAL NEEDS

MND affects many of the bodily functions, therefore, attention to the individual's need to be able to breathe, eat, drink, rest, communicate, express sexuality and obtain treatment for unpleasant symptoms and infections will be necessary before higher needs can be considered.

Dyspnoea

Most people with MND experience breathlessness at some time during their illness. This can be caused by weakening respiratory muscles, anxiety or a combination of the two. A calm, confident approach by the carer can greatly reduce anxiety in the patient and good ventilation in the room, either by opening windows or use of an electric fan, can also bring relief.

Severe feelings of breathlessness can be relieved by administration of opiate medication, such as diamorphine, which may be used if necessary over a long period of time without ill effect. Where opiate medication is used, an aperient containing a faecal softener and peristaltic stimulant should be used routinely to prevent constipation.

Home mechanical ventilation

Home mechanical ventilation (HMV) is rarely recommended for MND patients in the UK, although it is regularly considered in the USA. When its use is considered, thought must also be given to the location of patient care following intervention. In America, most people return home after their condition has been stabilized on a ventilator. Ventilation may be achieved by either:

- non-invasive ventilation by use of nasal/mouth intermittent positive pressure ventilator (used where patient is conscious, co-operative and has a good cough reflex);
- tracheostomy intermittent positive pressure ventilation (may be used where patient is in an emergency state of respiratory failure and is unable to cough).

Mechanical ventilation is not a procedure to be entered into lightly and, if considered, should be discussed well in advance of its need by patient, family and physician. In many cases it would be inappropriate and its use can cause much distress to patient and family if they are unaware of the full implications at the outset of treatment. Consideration should include the following points.

- Patient motivation. A high level of motivation is needed if mechanical ventilation is to succeed.
- Family motivation. The family must be able and willing to support home mechanical ventilation possibly for many years.
- Access to a consultant who is skilled in the use of mechanical ventilation and willing to provide support.

- Access to equipment necessary to support mechanical ventilation. Ventilators cost many hundreds of pounds per year in rental costs, which may have to be found by the patient and family.
- Physical and psychological suitability of the patient for this type of treatment. Not all MND patients experience life-threatening dyspnoea in the early stages of MND and, even if they do, many would be unable to accept this intervention psychologically.
- Care support in the home increases dramatically. If family and friends are unable to help, paid helpers could place an extreme financial burden on the patient and family.
- Experienced health professionals needed in addition to extra carers may not be available to help with care.

Oppenheimer (1993) concludes 'HMV can be a successful option for people with ALS (MND), but it should be reserved for selected highly motivated patients and families who can arrange the considerable resources, preparation, and caregiver support needed'. Initially, it may be argued that care should not be withheld because of financial restraints but, were this not the case, there would still be enormous physical and emotional pressures placed on the patient and family. It is arguable that at a time when the patient and family are already trying to live with significant life changes, a decision of this magnitude could be overwhelming.

Sleeping

Breathlessness is often noticed first during the night – a common cause being positioning of the patient. When sleeping in a horizontal position, gravity exerting pressure on the respiratory muscles can reduce the lung function. Many people find lying in a semi-reclined position, using pillows and/or a backrest, can ease their breathing.

It has been noted as the disease progresses that some patients cannot find a comfortable position in bed at all. This may be due to respiratory difficulties, but other factors may also be involved. The following case study illustrates this point.

Richard was 31 years old when he was diagnosed as having MND. As the disease progressed, he had great difficulty finding a position in bed where he felt able to breathe easily. As time went by, he spent less time in bed at night and more time sleeping sitting up in his wheelchair. Six months before his death, he ceased going to bed at all, and slept in his wheelchair at all times.

On discussion, Richard explained that he felt vulnerable lying in bed. He was unable to move, sit up or roll over and if his breathing became difficult, he could not use the call system easily, and knew there would be a time delay before anyone could help. Sitting in his chair, his breathing was easier and he felt he had more control over his environment.

The use of a reclining armchair with leg rest can be helpful in some cases; many people with MND find an electrically operated riser/recliner armchair helpful during the day. Some people spend the night in their armchair if they enjoy the independence of being able to change their position as often as they wish and mobility in bed is impaired.

Medication

It may be necessary to review medication being taken by the patient. Some medication prescribed for control of cramps and spasms can have a depressing effect on respiration, particularly large doses of diazepam. The benefits derived from the diazepam may need to be weighed against the detrimental effect this may be having on the respiration.

Chest infections

These may be experienced at any stage of the illness and may be caused by viral infection or aspiration of food or fluids. Weakened respiratory muscles reduce the efficiency of the cough which is the body's natural method of removing debris from the lungs.

Antibiotic medication should be prescribed, preferably at the first sign of an infection, and is usually successful in resolving the problem. Chest physiotherapy may be helpful if it can be tolerated by the patient.

Excess mucus and secretions caused by the infection may present a problem to the patient with weak respiratory muscles. Assisted coughing techniques can be used by the physiotherapist to help clear the chest, and can be taught to the carer for use at home.

Dysphagia

Difficulty in swallowing is a complex problem usually involving muscle weakness, spasticity and incoordination in the muscles of the mouth and throat. A detailed assessment by the speech and language therapist can help to identify the exact nature of the problem. A visit to a regional hospital may be suggested if facilities are not available locally to undertake specialized tests, which may be necessary to identify the problem.

Generally, anxiety can exacerbate an already difficult situation. A calm approach by the carer is most helpful. Attention should be given to preparation before mealtimes. Adequate time should be allowed and a relaxed atmosphere should be encouraged. If the meal is likely to take long enough for the food to get cold, the use of a plate warmer may be considered.

Types of food

Most people wish to continue eating 'normal' food for as long as possible. A dietitian or speech and language therapist can advise on the texture of foods most suitable for people with swallowing problems, and may also suggest ways of increasing calorie intake if problems become more severe.

Liquidized food usually appears most unappetizing and generally finely chopped or home minced lean meat (shop bought mince usually contains a high proportion of fat and creates a gritty texture when cooked) is easier to swallow and more palatable. Imaginative use of a cookery book can produce recipes for savoury and sweet souffles or mousses, which may be acceptable or adaptable.

Dehydration

Most people find that even-textured, semi-solid food is easier to swallow than liquid. Extra fluids can be added to the diet by the inclusion of ice cream, jelly, iced lollies, or fruit and vegetables such as melon or courgettes in the diet.

Food supplements are usually produced in liquid form but may be frozen either as ice cubes or in a block, if this is easier to swallow. It may be necessary to decant supplements if they are produced in a metal can or sufficient space is not left in the carton for expansion during freezing.

Positioning

The best position for eating is usually thought to be seated in a chair with an inclined back of about 15–20° from the upright, at a table of comfortable height for the patient. The head, shoulders and back should be supported; if the head is allowed to fall too far forward or backwards swallowing can be inhibited. This said, individual preferences vary and it is always wise to ask and experiment to find the most suitable position for each individual.

Aids to swallowing

Some people find that the application of ice externally to the throat (e.g. a bag of frozen peas) can help to encourage the swallowing reflex. Others have found that sucking crushed ice or an ice cube wrapped in gauze immediately prior to eating a meal has a similar effect. In addition, the speech and language therapist may be able to suggest exercises to maintain chewing and swallowing for as long as possible.

There is a variety of equipment available to help people to feed themselves. This can range from cutlery with padded handles and plate guards to mobile arm supports. The occupational therapist should be able to advise in this area.

Many people with MND are unable to clear food particles from their mouths after eating a meal. Thorough cleaning of the mouth following meals can improve patient comfort.

Saliva

Excess saliva can present a problem. The average adult produces about two litres of saliva a day (Bosma and Brodie, 1969) and, if swallowing is impaired for whatever reason, removal of excess saliva from the mouth will be necessary.

Medication in the form of atropine 0.6 mg three times a day may help, as can transdermal hyoscine. Side effects of some medication such as imipramine (50–20 mg *nocte*) produce a reduction in secretions and can have the added effect of lightening the mood of the patient.

It has been found that this type of medication can increase the viscosity of the saliva, making swallowing and breathing more of a problem and some people find the excess saliva preferable. If this is the case, a suction machine can be used to remove excess saliva (see p. 86).

Clothing

For people who experience the embarrassment of excess saliva, thought should be given to the type of clothing worn. The MNDA produce a range of leaflets on patient care, one of which focuses on this problem. Suggestions include garments with front panels backed with waterproof material and front panels which can be removed and replaced easily. Bibs should be avoided if possible, except at mealtimes, since they can cause great humiliation to the wearer.

Medication

Administration of medication can become a problem if swallowing is difficult. When prescribing medication, it is advisable to check with the patient and carer if there is a preferred form that the medication should take. Some people find tablets easier to swallow than liquid medication, even if their swallowing appears to be severely affected. It is helpful if the doctor checks this with the patient each time medication is prescribed, since this is an area that can change between visits.

Many types of medication can be obtained as tablet, capsule or syrup/liquid. Crushing tablets and mixing them with ice cream or prescribing medication to be administered as a suppository may be necessary if swallowing is particularly difficult.

Syringe drivers/subcutaneous infusion pumps

The use of a portable syringe driver or subcutaneous infusion pump may be considered if symptom control cannot be achieved with oral medication. This situation may be caused by weakness or exhaustion, severe swallowing problems or persistent, intractable symptoms. Medication can be given as a continuous subcutaneous infusion over 24 hours causing little problem to either patient or carer.

Syringe drivers are not confined to use in hospitals and can be set up and monitored in the home by the general practitioner and district nurse. Their use for controlling pain, nausea, vomiting, excess secretions and agitation is documented in the area of palliative care (Oliver, 1988). Whilst their use is more common in the later stages of the illness, they may also be used to good effect at an earlier stage, if necessary.

Choking

Coughing is a reflex action, used by the body to clear food or secretions from the bronchial tubes. Whilst coughing is still possible, the likelihood of death occurring by choking is very slight. A study by Saunders, Walsh and Smith in 1981 of 100 patients reported that only one patient died as a result of choking. It is, however, one of the major fears of many patients with MND and their carers that the patient will die during a choking attack.

Once again, the most constructive method of helping a person with MND who is experiencing a choking attack is to remain calm. These attacks often occur at mealtimes and may be triggered by hypersensitivity of the mouth or pharynx. It is important that helpers feel confident in their ability to help should an attack occur. Advice in this area may be given by the speech and language therapist or physiotherapist. Frequent attacks of choking require investigation and, in many cases, a solution can be suggested.

Assisted coughing

If the patient is seated or lying in a reclined position, it is helpful to bring them to the upright position. This places pressure beneath the diaphragm and improves the effect of coughing.

If the patient has enough strength and movement, he can be taught the technique of depressing the abdomen in time with the cough. This also increases the effects of the cough.

A physiotherapist or speech and language therapist will usually be able to teach the carer procedures designed to dislodge food particles, should the need arise. Ideas on the various techniques used may change, depending on current first aid procedures, and health professionals will need to update themselves as necessary on the most recent thinking.

Suction

In addition to removing excess saliva from the mouth and pharynx, suction machines can be used to clear food particles, particularly if a yankeur catheter is fitted. As chewing becomes more difficult, more attention will need to be given to mouth care. Suction can be useful for removing excess fluid/mouthwash following mouth care if the patient is unable to do this for himself.

Breathing space kit

This concept was developed by the MNDA to reduce the fears of people with MND and their carers. The breathing space kit enables patients and carers to have medication on hand at home to help relieve the stress of a choking attack.

Leaflets produced to accompany the kit are aimed at providing information for the patient, carer and professional carers. It is hoped that the leaflets will help to encourage discussion about the ultimate effects of the disease between patient, carer and professional carers. In this way, fears and anxieties can be reduced.

The medication suggested by the MNDA is in the form of three stesolid suppositories (10 mg) to be administered by the carer if necessary and three intramuscular injections of diamorphine (5 mg), hyoscine hydrobromide (0.4 mg/1 ml) and chlorpromazine (25 mg/1 ml), which can be administered by a doctor or nurse at the request of a doctor (see also Chapter 7).

In the event of a choking attack which does not resolve following normal procedures, the patient may become excessively breathless and be unable to regain his normal breathing pattern. The carer can administer a stesolid suppository to help relax the patient, and call the general practitioner for assistance. If the patient does not respond to the stesolid alone, intramuscular medication is on hand for the general practitioner to administer if required.

The breathing space kit can be used as a first aid measure without fear of harming the patient. The only lasting effect from the medication is positive, in that the injection acts as an amnesiac, so memories of the attack will be less distressing for the patient. The effects of the medication do not shorten a person's life.

Details of the breathing space kit and how it may be supplied for a named patient by a general practitioner can be obtained from the MNDA, on request.

Surgical interventions

Some patients find that saliva pools in the pharynx, which may result if the cricopharyngeus muscle tightens or some of the muscles in the throat become weaker. Fluid can then leak into the airways, which may cause persistent coughing or aspiration after taking food or drink, and may be irritating to the patient and carer.

There are two forms of surgical intervention – cricopharyngeal myotomy and parenteral feeding – which may be helpful in the management of this problem for people with MND. Neither will cure the illness but, if used appropriately, they can be effective methods of symptom control.

Cricopharyngeal myotomy

The cricopharyngeus muscle acts as a sphincter in the throat, helping to ensure that food and fluids pass into the oesophagus rather than into the lungs. If spastic paralysis is experienced related to MND, painless spasm of this muscle can prevent complete swallowing, resulting in pooling of food and fluids in the throat.

Norris, Smith and Denys (1985) describe their experience of surgical intervention and conclude that a clear selection procedure should be implemented. This is necessary to reduce the early experiences of major complications and treatment failures resulting from lack of careful screening.

Careful assessment is needed to ensure that the patient would be helped by this procedure. Many people with MND suffer from swallowing problems but few will be helped by this specific operation.

Parenteral feeding

In some instances, particularly when patients suffer from bulbar palsy, swallowing becomes laborious and exhausting. Patients may also suffer from frequent choking attacks associated with food and fluid intake, and the amount of nutrition they are able to take in by mouth does not fulfil their physical needs.

Over a period of time, the patient becomes dehydrated and malnourished which in turn can cause depression and increased weakness. This can lead to severe distress to the patient and carer alike, since the patient feels hungry and thirsty most of the time.

In this situation, it may be necessary to consider alternative methods of feeding. Newrick and Langton-Hewer (1984) observe that 'the profession's objective in the late stages of the disease is to minimise suffering and not simply to preserve life'. They feel that surgical intervention of this type is not appropriate. Norris, Smith and Denys (1985), however, observe 'Is it preferable to die of starvation and thirst, as well as amyotrophic lateral sclerosis (MND), because the attending doctors do not think "it right" to relieve the additional suffering?'

In practice, parenteral feeding is a form of symptomatic treatment which can, in some cases, improve the quality of life for patients with MND. The best interests of the patient must be borne in mind at all times, and it has been found that patients are usually prepared to make decisions for themselves, providing they are given the information they need.

If patients are experiencing severe hunger, thirst and weight loss there are few options open to the physician. If inability to swallow is experienced during the terminal stage of the illness, it is rarely accompanied by hunger and thirst, and administration of medication by syringe driver or injection is indicated to maintain the comfort of the patient.

Nasogastric tube feeding or gastrostomy appear to be the usual choice of alternative methods of feeding in Britain at present. Oesophagostomy or jejunostomy may also be considered, but the choice of surgical procedure depends to a large extent on the personal preferences of the individual surgeon involved.

Nasogastric tube

Nasogastric tube feeding carries low risks to the patient, in that it can be positioned without need of an anaesthetic. It can, however, cause irritation to the throat and is cosmetically more obvious. It may block more easily than a gastrostomy tube and so may require changing quite frequently, but this is a relatively simple procedure. Once the tube is sited, patients can be fed with high energy liquid feed instead of, or in addition to, the nourishment they can take by mouth.

Percutaneous endoscopic gastrostomy

A percutaneous endoscopic gastrostomy will usually require a general anaesthetic to site initially. It will need replacement after about nine months but this can be performed by local anaesthetic and usually the patient does not need an overnight stay at the hospital. The tube is inserted through the abdominal wall directly into the stomach. A small washer inside the stomach prevents the tube from coming loose.

The patient can then be fed with high energy liquid feed. It is usually recommended that this is done over a period of a few hours, possibly overnight, using an electrical pump. It is possible to 'bolus feed' using a catheter-tipped syringe but this is time consuming, and it has been found that patients tolerate the feed better if it is gradually introduced over a period of a few hours rather than by the bolus method.

The introduction of a gastrostomy catheter in no way interrupts the patient's ability to eat or drink if they are able, but it removes the pressure of having to try to take in all nutritional requirements by mouth.

Following a randomized study of patients with persistent neurological dysphagia in 1992, Park *et al.* concluded that 'percutaneous endoscopic gastrostomy tube feeding is a safe, effective and acceptable method of providing long term enteral nutrition in neurological patients'. If the prognosis is thought to be greater than four to six weeks, gastrostomy should be considered, whereas 'Nasogastric tube feeding should be used for only short term nutritional support'.

Counselling

Parenteral feeding for people with MND is surrounded by controversy, an example of which has already been cited. The decision as to whether a patient is considered for an alternative method of feeding is never easy. Time must be provided for explaining the procedures available and encouraging discussion with the patient and family about the issues involved and what is right for them.

The role of 'counsellor' may fall to any of the multidisciplinary team but information from the dietitian and/or gastric nurse should be sought. Through these discussions, it will usually become obvious as to the way forward, and it is important for the health professionals to be able to remain impartial throughout. The following case study gives an example of how the issues surrounding parenteral feeding may be addressed.

Bill was 64 years old and lived alone. He had begun to experience mild symptoms of bulbar palsy two years previously following the death of his mother. These had become progressively more severe as the illness progressed and resulted in loss of intelligible speech, severe swallowing difficulties of food, fluid and saliva, and weakness of the shoulder girdle and upper arms. His mobility was good and he could still perform most activities of daily living independently.

He began attending the day unit at the local palliative care unit once a week to provide social contact and symptom control following referral from his general practitioner. His main concern at this time was of excess saliva and difficulty in chewing, which he felt sure were due to his ill-fitting dentures.

Through the following three months, the excess saliva continued to cause difficulties and did not respond to any medication. Despite various alterations to his dentures, Bill's chewing and swallowing continued to deteriorate and at this time, it was also noticed that he looked to be losing weight and was becoming more tired. He was having great difficulty swallowing food or liquid at the day unit but insisted that he was eating well at home. This was difficult to disprove since he lived alone.

Following considerable concern voiced by all members of the team, Bill was offered admission to the palliative care unit, for observation, to discover if anything could be done to improve his swallowing and prevent further weight loss. On admission, he weighed eight stones four pounds, a loss of three stones since the beginning of his illness two years previously. He could only manage to eat a small amount of ice cream and some cornflakes with milk, and had two major choking attacks which required suction to resolve in the space of four days. He could swallow very little fluid or his medication, either in tablet form or syrup.

Bill was examined by the consultant and was found to be in reasonably good health apart from his swallowing problems and, following discussion with the team, it was decided to offer the option of parenteral feeding. Bill communicated by pen and paper, so conversations were lengthy, but it was ascertained that he felt hungry and thirsty all of the time. He was most reluctant to admit that he could not eat or drink – this was only made possible by his stay on the unit, where he was unable to deny his problems.

Once the problem had been established, it was suggested to him that there were procedures that, whilst they could not cure his condition, could stop him from feeling hungry and thirsty and improve his energy levels.

Nasogastric feeding and gastrostomies were explained to him (being the usual procedures used in the area) and questions about the risks, whether he would be able to continue to live at home and the extra help he may need were answered honestly. This discussion also provided an opportunity to talk about Bill's life and death which had not been possible before. After this, he felt he needed some time to consider the information he had been given, and discuss it with a close friend.

The following day he made the decision to go ahead with the operation to perform a gastrostomy, providing the surgeon and anaesthetist felt he would be suitable for a general anaesthetic. He was transferred to the local general hospital where the operation was performed and he returned to the unit two days later.

He was visited by the dietitian and gastric nurse and it was decided that he would be fed by electric pump overnight. Once this had been established, Bill returned home with support from the district nurses, social services home helps and his warden. He increased attendance at the day unit to two days and was visited regularly by the dietitian to monitor his food intake and weight.

The main problem that was experienced was that since Bill was quite mobile, a careful check had to be made on his weight. His calorie intake had to be increased to take this mobility into account, and it was also necessary to add in a bolus feed during the day as he still felt hungry.

Bill continued to eat small amounts of food for a few weeks but found the choking attacks he experienced were frightening. He also had difficulty accepting that he was being fed, because the food was not passing through his mouth.

His quality of life improved to the extent that he continued to gain weight slowly, had more energy and was not permanently hungry and thirsty. He was able to join in with activities and outings at the day unit and continue to live at home with the support of his friends and health professionals.

Bowel regularity

MND does not affect sphincter muscles and patients do not become incontinent of urine or faeces. Poor abdominal muscle control and altered food and fluid intake can, however, cause changes in bowel habit. Care should be taken that, however little the patient appears to be eating or drinking, their bowels move at least once every three to four days.

A dietitian can advise on fibre-rich foods, bulking agents or ways to improve fluid intake but this may be insufficient to promote regular bowel action. Aperient medication in the form of a faecal softener (e.g. lactulose) and peristaltic stimulant (e.g. senna), or a combined preparation (co-danthramer or co-danthrusate) may be necessary to resolve the problem.

Insomnia

There can be various reasons why a person has difficulty sleeping and it will be necessary to discover the cause before treating accordingly. The most common reasons for insomnia in MND are listed below.

Dyspnoea

Discomfort of any kind can cause sleeping problems. An inability to breathe or fears relating to the ease of breathing can be a cause of insomnia (see p.80).

Pain

Careful attention to pressure-relieving mattresses, positioning and regular turning can reduce pain. Opiate medication (MST® 10 mg *nocte*) can help to relieve the general pain of immobility (see Chapter 5).

Fear

Some people feel vulnerable in bed as their mobility, ability to communicate or summon assistance is reduced. They may also fear that they will not wake up if they go to sleep.

As has been said, attention should be given to expressing these fears and trying to reassure the patient where possible. Touch-sensitive buzzers can be made cheaply to enable help to be summoned and, with the aid of the speech and language therapist if necessary, a form of non-verbal communication may be developed.

Cat napping

Short periods of sleep during the day can reduce the ability to sleep at night. Benzodiazepine medication such as temazepam (10–12 mg) can be helpful in establishing a good sleep pattern.

Cramps and spasms

Cramps can be particularly troublesome at night. Quinine (300–600 mg) may be used or diazepam (5–10 mg *nocte*), which acts as a muscle relaxant and has the added effect of causing drowsiness.

If spasms are a general problem, baclofen 5 mg three times a day increased to 30–60 mg daily (maximum 100 mg daily) or dantrolene 25 mg daily which can be increased to a maximum 400 mg daily may be used. Whilst severe spasm can be painful, overmedication can result in flaccidity which can cause difficulty for the carer when transferring the patient.

Dysarthria

It is thought that between 75–80% of people with MND will experience some difficulty with speech during the progression of their illness. The speech and language therapist should be involved as soon as any alterations in speech are noticed. Whilst she cannot prevent the ultimate deterioration of a person's speech, there are many strategies which may be used to prolong functional speech.

Communication equipment

Communication can be maintained in some form, however basic, throughout the course of the illness if this is the wish of the patient. Experience has found that as many as five or six communication aids may be needed by an individual patient during the progression of the illness (Langton-Hewer, 1988).

Computers

The advent of the microchip and the use of computers and computerized speech synthesizers has revolutionized the field of communication aids. Computerized equipment, however, is expensive to provide and needs specialized assessment by the speech and language therapist or centre for human communication to ensure the user is provided with the equipment most suited to their needs.

Where an assessment for a computer to aid with communication is recommended, it will be necessary to ascertain whether funding is available to provide the equipment suggested through the health authority or if funding will need to be obtained independently. Care should be taken not to raise a person's hopes of obtaining expensive equipment if funding is not available. However, most assessment centres require that agreement of funding be obtained before the assessment can be undertaken.

Computers and speech synthesizers have improved communication for many people with MND since they can be used with microswitches, activated by very small but reliable movements of any part of the body. It is not yet possible, however, to enable a person to communicate with the speed and efficiency of normal speech. At the time of writing, initial tests are being carried out on computers activated by brain waves which, if successful, could be an important development for people with MND.

Electronic communication aids

Computers can be used for communication by speech and writing (if attached to a printer) but, for many people, a small portable easy-to-use device is more appropriate. The double-sided LCD displays featured on the Lightwriter range of communicators (Toby Churchill, Cambridge, England) enable efficient communication with another individual and within a group of people. It can be accessed from a typewriter-style keyboard (on the more basic models) or by a switch-operated scanning screen (on the later models).

In addition, new electronic communication aids are being developed by other manufacturers. A speech and language therapist will be able to help in the assessment and recommendation of equipment suitable to the needs of the individual.

Mechanical communication equipment

Other forms of communication such as an alphabet card, eye pointing frame or pen and paper may be found to be quicker than a computer when holding a conversation with another person. Perspex eye pointing frames have the advantage of face-to-face communication and constant eye contact. They are quicker than computers and hold the listener's attention. They are cheap and simple to make and can be customized to the individual's needs as necessary. They do not require electricity and are easily transported. They require the minimum amount of user movement – letters are identified by patients pointing to them with their eyes, a movement which is rarely lost by people with MND.

As with any communication aid, this form of communication can be tiring – particularly to the 'listener'. Speech is quicker than any equipment and most people will persevere with speech until they are unable to make themselves understood before resorting to any equipment. It is, therefore, important that the patient becomes familiar with any equipment before it becomes essential.

Sexuality

A patient's sexuality does not end with the diagnosis of terminal illness.
(Kaye, 1991).

'Sexuality is a normal part of being human' (Mearns and Thorne, 1992). It is linked to all aspects of a person's life, not only their sex life (Webb, 1985). In the early stages of MND, physical disability is usually minimal. It is unlikely, therefore, to affect a person's physical relationship with their partner. Common areas of concern at this stage usually centre around sexual transmission of the illness to the partner, the risk of transmission should a pregnancy result, or whether sexual intercourse could accelerate the course of the disease.

MND is not sexually transmitted and the progression of the illness is not affected by sexual intercourse. In a small number of cases (*c.* 5–10%), there is a clear family history of MND. At the time of diagnosis a family history is obtained and, if a family link is discovered, genetic counselling may be considered to evaluate the risks involved for the family members concerned.

As the illness progresses, the patient may need his partner to take a more active/dominant role. SPOD (The Association to Aid Sexual and

Personal Relationships of People with Disability) provide advice and practical suggestions, as well as a counselling service for people with disabilities.

Sexual concerns are not easily discussed by many health professionals with their patients. It is rare for a doctor or nurse to take a sexual history but if questions are phrased with sensitivity, for example 'How does this illness affect your relationship?', the patient is given an opportunity to discuss the matter further, if wished.

The following sections list some areas where difficulties may occur.

Body image

Physical appearances are more important to some people than to others. MND does not always affect a person's physical appearance dramatically but changes do take place.

Muscle wasting, problems with excess saliva or the need to use splints, head supports or the like alter a person's body image. In addition, the partner may find these changes difficult to accept. The underlying feelings of the partner towards the patient may remain unchanged, but they may feel frightened or anxious by this unattractiveness, and find this issue difficult to admit and accept.

Weakness and tiredness

People with MND often become weak and tired during the progression of the illness. They may just not have the energy needed to enjoy sexual intercourse. In addition, they may experience pain from increasingly immobile joints and the partner may fear hurting them, when held or cuddled.

Privacy

This may be a problem as the illness progresses. The number of people involved in looking after a person with MND in the home can become extensive and a normally quiet home can be turned into a constant round of people coming in to help. It may be necessary to look at ways in which some times of the day are kept free of visitors, to enable the patient and family to have time on their own.

If a person is cared for in hospital or a nursing home, privacy can be scarce. Some hospitals and nursing homes acknowledge the need for patient privacy, but many need reminding of the needs of the patient and family. Couples need undisturbed time together and it is important that they feel able to ask for this if necessary.

Communication

Actions speak louder than words – and they tell the truth.
(Barney, 1993).

Honest communication between a couple facing MND is vital. People need to give and receive love even if they are too ill to express this in a sexual way. Intimacy, closeness and touch are very important, particularly to those who may feel themselves to be untouchable, useless and unlovable. A hug or a cuddle can sometimes help a great deal.

As the patient becomes less mobile, the carer's role will become more demanding; for example, the patient may ask to be repositioned frequently. This may be a way of asking for physical contact and the manner in which the carer responds carries a powerful message to the patient. Taking a little extra care can help patients feel that they are still acceptable people.

Infections

As has been said, general infections should be treated with appropriate antibiotic medication, preferably before the patient becomes severely symptomatic.

Dry, sore eyes may be a complication of MND and seem to be the result of decreased blinking. Hypromelose eye drops can lubricate the eye, but an antibiotic preparation will be needed to resolve an infection. Drops may cause smarting or stinging and eye ointment may be preferred by the patient.

Mouth infections can result as chewing and movement of the mouth are reduced. The most common is candidiasis (thrush) which can be treated with nystatin® or ketaconozole. Good oral hygiene can reduce the occurrence of mouth infections.

As the person with MND becomes weaker, resistance to infection lowers. Prompt attention to infections can reduce discomfort and help to maintain good general health.

SAFETY AND SECURITY

Once physiological needs have been addressed, a person needs to have a safe, secure base from which to operate. Physical safety in the form of suitable housing, protection from danger and the ability to control the environment in which the patient lives will need attention. In addition psychological factors encompassing the maintenance of routines, management of changes to that routine, and the perceived effects the illness is exacting upon the family can also affect the patient's feelings of safety and security.

Physical issues

Caring for a person with MND at home can be emotionally and physically exhausting, particularly as the level of disability becomes more severe. The carer gradually realizes that she is living life for two people in the time, and often with the resources, available for one.

Although we were told at the time of diagnosis how the illness would affect *J* and how it would end, we didn't really understand the full implications of what was being said. It was probably as well really.

I thought I could manage on my own but I realize now that I need help.

These statements were made by the wives of two men who had been living with MND for over a year. They managed well with minimal help until the restrictions of the illness began to change their lives dramatically. Neither were young women, but both managed to care for their husbands, with appropriate support, for the greater part of their illness.

Attention to the physical environment is often necessary at an early stage of the illness. Many homes do not lend themselves to use by a severely disabled person and may need adaptation to provide a safe environment for the patient. Provision of hand rails, stairlifts, level access shower and toilet units and ramps, or the building of extensions, are the province of the occupational therapist, who will need to assess the home situation for possible alterations well in advance of the need for their use.

Environmental control systems (see Chapter 4) can also help to improve the patient's feelings of safety and security. Despite severe disability, it can still be possible for the patient to control elements of the environment as diverse as turning lights on and off, making a phone call or opening the door.

Involvement of the multidisciplinary team often implies team members visiting and providing support within the home. In addition, there are ways in which outside help and support can be given, whilst still enabling patients to be cared for in their own home for most of the time.

Day care

Provision of day care varies with the age and ability of the patient and the area in which they live. Some elderly people's homes, hospitals and nursing homes offer day care, as do young physically disabled units or centres.

Increasingly, hospices and palliative care units recognize the benefits of providing day care facilities for their patients. Some are also willing to offer day care to people with MND. Whilst many hospices and palliative care units would like to be able to offer more care to people with MND, their resources may only allow for provision of day care or home care support.

Day care can provide an opportunity for the patient and carer to have a break from each other's company. Relationships may suffer extreme pressure once the patient is no longer able to work or leave the house on his own, particularly if he is unable to be left alone whilst the carer is out of the house. It can be pleasant to spend time with a loved one from choice, but if the freedom of choice is removed, tensions can place undue strain on the relationship.

Day care arranged for a set day or days during the week allows for the carer to plan outings and appointments. This usually provides the carer with a longer period of time than would be possible if a sitter came into the home.

Many day centres can offer personal care in the form of bathing or hair dressing and social activities. Some may have medical, occupational therapy and physiotherapy support as well. Day care can help patients to develop new interests and provide added conversation topics on their return home.

Many people with MND feel isolated at home as their mobility decreases. Many carers find this difficult to understand, as they are often willing to take the patient out but these offers are refused. Bob explained his reluctance to go out following deterioration of his physical condition: 'The first time you go to a new place in a wheelchair is difficult. It takes a lot of courage to get over this'.

Many people have difficulty accepting that they are dependent on others for mobility. This can be of particular significance if driving and independence of mobility have been of great importance to them in the past. Attending a day unit helped Bob to meet new people in a similar situation to his own. This did not make going to new places any easier but it gave him the incentive to try. Attendance at the day centre also gave his wife a break each week, which helped her to continue caring for him at home (see also Chapter 4).

Respite care

Day care can help relieve the pressures of caring week by week but occasionally the carer may need a longer break. This may become necessary if the patient becomes severely disabled and the carer becomes tired or unwell and is unable to care for the patient at home. The carer may also have other family commitments or need a longer break than a day or two during the week.

Requests for respite care often carry additional messages and this aspect should be explored. Relieving the carer of their burden by arranging respite care may seem to be the answer. It can, however, result in more problems for the carer who, having had the burden lifted, is reluctant to return to the caring role once again.

Many people experience difficulty in asking for help, and asking for respite care may be the way in which the carer asks for more help in the home, more emotional support or to say she has reached the stage where care at home is no longer possible in her eyes. Provision of respite care, without looking at the whole care package, can lead to a breakdown on the patient's return home.

The progression of MND may be accompanied by unpleasant symptoms. Whilst the illness cannot be cured, in many cases symptoms can be controlled. For example, excessive tiredness on the part of the patient and carer may result from pain or spasm, preventing sleep.

Hicks and Corcoran (1993) suggest that ' "Respite care" is a much misunderstood term'. They feel that respite care could and should offer the opportunity to review symptom control and community care, in addition to providing a break for the carer. They conclude that 'patients with MND have much to gain from respite admissions to hospices and that these facilities should be more widely available'.

If a keyworker is involved, they will probably have an idea of the problems facing the patient and family and may be able to work towards resolution of these problems in the community, before a crisis is reached. If not, admission to a hospice can give the opportunity to explore the problems and work towards their solution.

Respite care may be sought in residential homes or specialist units as well as in hospices/palliative care units. Few, if any, hospitals are now able to offer respite care facilities, and the introduction of the community care provision places a greater emphasis on care being undertaken by private nursing/residential homes.

Assessments for suitability for respite care in residential homes may be undertaken by care managers. Referral can be made through the local social services department or directly to care management and will usually be followed by the care manager contacting the patient and family to arrange a visit. This will involve discussion about existing care and a financial assessment. The care manager may also require assessments from health professionals already involved in provision of care for the patient.

Once this information has been received, the care manager will be able to advise the patient and family of any help they can be offered in financing respite care. They will also be able to help with finding a suitable nursing/residential home to undertake the care.

Most people with MND wish to be cared for in their own homes and, following adequate discussion, usually accept that help will need to be sought to enable this to happen safely. It is important that these issues are discussed early in the progression of the illness and that carers are encouraged to accept help before they become tired and entrenched in their duties.

Psychological issues

Routine and familiarity help to promote feelings of safety and security. As the illness progresses, a person with MND will have to address many changes in routine, and the way in which this is handled will affect the way in which the patient copes with these changes.

The most basic change of routine will occur if the patient has been employed in work away from the home. As the illness progresses, they may not be able to continue as before and despite alterations to the working pattern, may need to give up work altogether. Discussion with the patient and carer as to the implications and the way in which the change will be addressed can be a positive step towards developing a new routine.

Health professionals can help to maintain routines by arranging to visit at times that are acceptable to the patient and family. This may be difficult initially but, as time and the illness progress, the routine of the health professional can usually be adjusted to meet the need.

As has been stated, a time may come when despite all efforts, the patient may not be able to be cared for at home. Accommodation may become unsuitable as the patient becomes more disabled, symptoms may become too severe or the carer may be unable to provide support for physical or emotional reasons.

This situation rarely arises suddenly and, if possible, should be discussed between the patient and carer before crisis point is reached. It may develop as a natural progression from respite care or may be necessary during the terminal phase of the illness if the carer feels unable to cope with this at home. However the situation arises, it will cause a major change in routine and will usually precipitate powerful emotions on the part of both patient and carer. The following case study illustrates this point.

> Bill had been living at home with his wife, Kitty, for two and a half years following his diagnosis of MND. Bill was in his early sixties and his wife was some six years older. They had been rehoused into a purpose-built, disabled person's bungalow and had managed at home with nursing and occupational therapy support.
>
> Bill attended the day unit at the local palliative care unit. He had developed a pattern of being admitted to the unit for two weeks' respite care (about 3–4 times a year) at his and his wife's request. As his illness had progressed, he and his wife began to experience more difficulties.
>
> They had discussed the possibility that Kitty would not be able to

care for Bill at home until his death, and both were in agreement that he would be cared for in a nursing home if the need arose. Kitty suffered from arthritis and lifting and transfers became a problem, particularly since Bill needed frequent positional changes and toileting requirements.

Despite the forward planning, Kitty had great difficulty in accepting that she could not care for Bill at home any longer. She became physically unwell and joint pains and recurrent viral infections finally helped Kitty to realize that Bill would have to go into residential care.

Through this time, Kitty received a great deal of help and support to overcome the guilt she felt at having to 'give in' to her own needs, the anger she felt towards the illness, and acceptance that she now had limitations of her own.

Arrangements were made for Bill to move to a nursing home where he stayed for the last year of his life. Kitty was able to help care for Bill in the nursing home, without the strain of lifting and attending to Bill's physical needs.

The difficulties arising from this change for both patient and carer can be reduced by visits to the new home before a final decision is made. Many patients are unaware of the strain they place upon their carer and may have difficulty in accepting the need that they be cared for elsewhere. Short stays prior to the permanent move can give staff and patient the opportunity to get to know each other and understand specific problems experienced by the patient.

The effects of MND can cause the patient to feel very vulnerable. Difficulty in communication through impaired speech, and the need to explain individual requirements to different members of staff can be most frustrating for the patient. Good communication between staff members is vital to prevent the patient suffering pain, anxiety and fear.

Family and friends can be less than helpful if the move to a nursing home becomes necessary. They are rarely closely involved and may voice doubts about the necessity for such drastic action. Individuals can cope with a finite amount of physical and emotional stress, and it is rare for the decision for the patient to move to a nursing home or the like to be reached without heart searching on both sides. A great deal of support is usually necessary for both patient and carer before, during and after the move.

The effects of MND on the patient and family are often seen to be physical. As the nerves die, the muscles are less able to respond to the signals transmitted by the brain since the motor pathways are incomplete. The psychological implications, however, are far more extensive than may be initially apparent. For example, introduction of equipment to aid independence can be rejected unless its arrival is timed correctly. Equipment that arrives too early will be rejected as it is not needed and challenges the sufferer to look at possible problems in the future. If it is too late, the patient will be unable to benefit by its use.

People with MND may also fear that the effects of their illness will become impossible for their family to bear. In their eyes, this may result in their being deserted by the people to whom they are closest. Reassurance from the carer may be needed to maintain security for the patient, and support will be needed for carers to ensure that they are able to continue in their role.

Empathetic understanding of problems by health professionals will greatly improve their ability to provide effective care whilst working with people suffering from MND and their families.

LOVE AND BELONGING

If people feel physiologically comfortable and safe and secure within their environment, social issues and those surrounding love and belonging will then become most important to them. How people view themselves in relation to family, friends and peer group, and their ability to give and receive love will need to be considered. This will include their changing role within the family and the team of people helping them, their need to remain productive, and their plans for the future.

Role changes

Most people adopt a variety of roles associated with their lifestyle, and either the roles or certain functions within them are constantly changing. This can be illustrated most easily by the role of motherhood which begins with the birth or adoption of a baby – at that time requiring the mother to give her full attention to the baby for the first few weeks of its life.

As the baby grows, the mother may have to return to employment outside the home, which will require that she delegates part of the function of being a mother to a child minder or nursery, whilst still maintaining the role of mother. This process is repeated throughout the time that the child is growing up through different situations. Once the child has reached adulthood and moved away from home, the nature of the role of mother will change once more.

A person with MND will still maintain the role of spouse, parent, sibling or child, but declining capabilities may mean that some of the functions within those roles may need to be delegated. Problems usually occur as a result of lack of choice in this area. A healthy person making a conscious decision to delegate certain functions within a role is very different from that person relinquishing them through ill health, probably against their wishes.

Some of the areas which may give rise to problems are listed in the next section.

Independence

Most people value independence more than they realize: it is a state which is often taken for granted. When one member of the family suffers from a degenerative illness like MND, that individual's decreasing independence threatens not only their roles within the family, but also the various roles that each family member assumes.

Gradually during the progression of the illness, the carer undertakes different functions that the patient can no longer perform, which can result in the patient feeling he has little left to contribute. The main carer may then feel weighed down by extra responsibilities. Intellect and memory are not affected by this illness and it is important to help the patient and family to adjust their thinking, enabling the patient to retain his role within the family, by encouraging him to retain as many of the functions as he feels able.

Dependence

As the muscles weaken, different abilities may be affected. Many people seem to equate speech problems with hearing loss and learning disability. It is not unusual for people with MND to be shouted at or spoken to in words of one syllable. Carers can become weary of explaining that this illness does not affect the intellect or memory. Society is becoming more aware of the needs of people living with disabilities, but may still view them with a certain amount of suspicion. Since people with MND rarely feel ill they do not place themselves easily into the sick role.

In certain situations, it may not be possible for the patient to continue as before and the action taken by the carer may help to reduce anxiety. This is illustrated in the following case study.

Tony had become too disabled with MND for his wife, Jane, to care for him at home. He was admitted to the local hospice from his home in a village some distance from the hospice. Jane was still living at home which meant her having to ask for lifts to visit Tony, since she was unable to drive.

Jane had reluctantly taken driving lessons in the past but the new situation provided the impetus to get more practice and apply to take her test. She was very nervous and lacked confidence in her abilities as a driver, but once she had passed her test both she and Tony were very relieved. Whilst Tony had been happy to be the sole driver before, he now felt pleased that Jane had increased her skills and was better prepared for life after his death.

Intimacy

When a wife or husband becomes carer to their spouse, the role of spouse itself often takes second place to that of nurse. This seems to happen imperceptibly, but as the illness progresses and more care is needed, the role of carer may overshadow the role of spouse. The following case study illustrates this point.

> Celia had cared for Barry at home since his diagnosis. Over a period of 15 months, he had become progressively more disabled. He was admitted to the local hospice during an episode of severe spasms, for symptom control. The spasms proved to be difficult to control and only became manageable after many weeks.
>
> By the time the spasms were controlled, Barry's mobility had decreased beyond the point that Celia felt she could manage at home. It was decided that he should remain at the hospice where he died, peacefully, six months later.
>
> Gradually, during those six months, Barry and Celia regained their relationship of husband and wife. They both felt they had lost this relationship during the progression of the illness prior to Barry's admission to the hospice. Relieving Celia of the need to nurse Barry allowed them the space they needed to regain their previous relationship, which was very precious to them both.

Many people wish and are able to care for their relatives at home. This, however, is not always the case, and it is possible to love someone very deeply but still be unable to look after their physical needs.

Adjusting to role changes

The effects of MND are rarely sudden: they become apparent over a period of weeks or maybe months. The change in roles occurs correspondingly slowly and may not be felt until a situation arises where the sufferer and carer are forced to face the change.

People react in various ways to these changes. The way in which they react will depend to a great extent on their basic personality and they way in which they have adjusted to changes in the past. Anger, anxiety or depression may be felt and problems can occur when a person has difficulty focusing these emotions appropriately, sharing them with the family and working towards a resolution.

Anger

Many people respond with anger to the possibility of change, particularly if it is brought about by circumstances beyond their control. Difficulties may arise if the patient cannot find an appropriate focus for anger and this may then result in it being transferred away from the original object of that anger. The following case study illustrates this point.

> Steve was 36 years old when MND was diagnosed. He was married to Mandy and they had three daughters under the age of 10. Steve had always made the decisions within the family until the effects of his illness caused severe problems to his mobility and his ability to care for himself. Mandy worked hard to enable Steve to continue to make decisions wherever possible, but this was not always practical.
>
> As the illness progressed, Steve became totally dependent on Mandy for his care and, whilst he was aware of his dependence, he became very anxious when she was not there for any reason. He was reluctant to look at what was happening to him as a result of his illness and, instead, exhibited anger towards Mandy and her ability to care for him.
>
> The anger became particularly passionate if she had to make a decision that he felt he would normally take, and this often resulted in his making unrealistic requests about his care or where this care should be obtained. Fierce verbal exchanges ensued and whilst this seemed to provide Steve with an outlet for his anger, Mandy felt hurt and unsure of future actions.

Anger can be a frightening emotion to experience whether it be within oneself or received from another. Whilst it is important to discuss matters surrounding the episode, it may be too much of a risk for the couple involved to look at this on their own. It can be constructive for an impartial outsider to help the people involved to explore what is occurring and how they may manage it in the future.

Depression

Depression may result from an inability to discuss worries and anxieties, or if the patient and family feel unsupported during the course of the illness. If it occurs, it often suggests that there are unsolved problems (Stedeford, 1984). On occasion, anti-depressant medication may be indicated by the diagnosis of a clinical depression but, whether or not anti-depressant medication is prescribed, time should be taken to explore possible problems and help towards their resolution.

Reactions to decreasing ability and mobility vary and are not always predictable, as the following case study shows.

James was referred for assessment after he had been diagnosed as having MND. His mobility was decreasing and this was beginning to cause problems with activities of daily living in the cottage where he lived with his wife and daughter, and at the offices where he ran his business.

At the initial assessment, his wife showed my colleague and myself around the house on her own and during this time expressed the view that her husband would not be able to tolerate living with MND and would probably take his own life. In the interview that followed with James and his wife, it became obvious that there were many problems to be faced. Living in a listed cottage caused problems when considering adaptations, but the most important issues related to future plans for the family.

James certainly had problems adjusting to his declining abilities, but with help and support both he and his wife were able to address many of these problems and plan for the future. They were, in fact, able to use the months of the progression of his illness constructively.

Social and leisure activities

Social and leisure activities will often assume more importance as the patient's physical ability decreases and he has more time available. Some people will be highly motivated to maintain an interest in hobbies, even if this entails adapting a physically orientated activity, such as participating in sport, into spectating as the person becomes less mobile. Other people find that alterations in their physical appearance and the need to use a wheelchair discourage them from maintaining social contact.

As the disease progresses, maintaining some form of social contact is necessary to prevent isolation, but it may be difficult. Visitors may become less frequent if the patient's physical appearance changes or communication becomes difficult. The use of computers can improve written communication in the form of letters, poems, stories or diaries and can be a useful way to maintain contact as the patient becomes weaker and is less able to leave the house.

ESTEEM AND SELF-REGARD

Each individual has a concept of himself comprising self-image (the person's perception of himself), self-esteem (the extent to which the person likes himself) and the ideal self (the person he would like to be). The level of a person's self-esteem is generally thought to be related to the perception of differences between that person's self-image and his ideal self. The esteem in which a person is held by others also contributes to his level of self-esteem.

Living with MND precipitates an ever-enlarging gap between the person's self-image and their ideal self. MND has been described as a disease of losses and this requires that both the person with the illness and the family live with an ever-changing situation in which the main changes relate to loss.

Whether we experience it or not, grief accompanies all the major changes in our lives.

(Tatelbaum, 1981).

People experience losses, even if the change is a positive one like a promotion at work or a new baby in the family. Acknowledgement of the losses that accompany change can allow for exploration, grieving and resolution to occur.

Assumptions can easily be made when working with someone who has MND. Loss of a person's life is usually thought to be the ultimate fear, but losses in other areas can be of more immediate significance to people with MND. Such losses may include loss of independence, mobility, control over their lives, freedom, role, employment, family or home, and should be considered as an integral part of offering care to this patient group.

Leick and Davidson-Neilsen (1987) identify four tasks related to grief work associated with life-threatening illness. These tasks can be seen to relate to the tasks of grieving identified by Worden (Chapter 8), and whilst this approach is not definitive, it is certainly worth consideration.

- *Task 1* Recognition of the consequences of the illness, the ability to make the illness real.
- *Task 2* Acknowledgement of the emotions surrounding the illness. These may include anger at the limitations placed upon the person or grief at the possibility of not seeing one's children reach maturity.
- *Task 3* Development of skills needed to live with the illness, the ability to reorganize thinking to meet the changing situation.
- *Task 4* Working to use energy for living in the present rather than worrying about the future.

People facing the losses associated with life-threatening illness need help and support in order to work towards enjoyment of life. Judy Tatelbaum quotes the work of Carl and Stephanie Simonton in her book, *The Courage to Grieve*. They recognize the importance of a well-developed support system for dealing with life crises and suggest the following:

    25% self-support
    20% spouse support
    55% environmental support

Large, extended families are less common in today's society, which leads to heavy reliance upon close family members. This appears to discourage the development of close friendships, the main component of wider environmental support systems. Equally, it is easy to overlook the importance of caring for ourselves, and expanding our inner resources. People rarely give thought to their support networks until a crisis occurs.

As a result of these factors, it often falls to the health professionals working with a family to provide the support needed, to work through the emotions surrounding the losses imposed upon the patient and family by the illness. It may be possible for health professionals to encourage widening of the family support network, but there may be a reluctance on the part of the family to do this. A co-ordinated team approach may be necessary to support an individual team member upon whom the family rely.

As the patient becomes weaker, it may be more difficult for them to see a purpose in life. Physical productivity may become impossible because of increasing immobility, but through attention to communication the patient can still contribute thoughts, reminiscences, stories, articles or, in some cases, books. Much depends on the personality and determination of the person concerned.

SELF-ACTUALIZATION

Rogers based his work on the belief that the discrepancy between a person's self-image and their ideal self can be reduced, and their self-esteem enhanced, by providing an environment of unconditional positive regard. Through this environment it is possible to grow towards self-actualization.

Attention to the issues surrounding physiological needs, safety and security, love and belonging and self-esteem can free people to become themselves and develop their potential. Self-actualization is usually a transient state and will be different for each individual – 'What a man **can** be, he **must** be' (Maslow, 1968). It may seem surprising that anyone living with a progressive neuromuscular disease could grow and develop but it is possible for the patient and/or carer to achieve a high degree of harmony between or within themselves.

SUMMARY OF NEEDS

The needs of the patient and carer at this stage of the disease can be summarized in three sections.

Maintain independence

> Being told the disease was a progressive one enabled me to do things while I could and not leave them in the hope that I would soon be feeling better.
>
> *(Henke, 1968).*

Much that has been written on this subject reinforces the view that people should make the most of their abilities whilst they are able to do so. Obviously, where possible this is sound advice but, in practice, it is often difficult for the patient to act upon it.

The speed of progression of the illness often involves the patient in much emotional adjustment and little time is left for getting out and about. Many patients and carers have voiced the opinion that 'we were only just beginning to come to terms with one aspect of this illness before we were forced to face another'; this may have a bearing on their ability to cope.

> Anticipation of needs before they become necessities is most important.
>
> *(Woodcock, 1985).*

Maintaining independence hinges upon this statement. It is impossible to prevent the slow deterioration, but intelligent anticipation of needs can lead to provision of advice and equipment. This helps to improve quality of life by enabling the patient to maintain the best level of function at each stage of the illness.

In order that the patient and carer are able to take advantage of the time available, they will need support from those around them. This involves family, friends and health professionals alike, working together to provide the encouragement and physical help and skills that will be necessary.

> The patient knows he is getting worse so the months become chapters of a horror novel·... Fellow patients, I challenge you to fight ... with all your might. To be successful you will need all the support you can get from the caring others in your environment.
>
> *(Woodcock, 1985).*

Emotional support

> Everything about the disease is certain to reduce your physical and emotional power. The emotional is much more difficult to cope with than the physical.
>
> *(Woodcock, 1985).*

> People don't realize the emotional implications of this disease, they see it as a physical illness.
>
> *(Paul Whiting, 1993).*

The progression of MND is unpredictable and the patient will need the help of various health professionals at different stages of the illness. There will be times when each of the health professionals involved in the care of the patient will wonder if their contribution is really necessary at that time.

It is often difficult for the patient and carer to acknowledge the benefits of help they receive during the progression of the illness; this may only be recognized after the death of the patient. Experience shows that throughout the illness it is important to maintain contact with the family to lend emotional support. Knowing that people care and can provide help when necessary can be most reassuring for the patient and family.

Quality of life

Surprisingly, there is some. The extent and degree depend on the patient.

(Woodcock, 1985).

I know that in the past five and a half years I have learnt more about life and the importance of the quality of human relationships than I had learnt in all the preceding years.

(Pollard, 1984).

Boredom is probably the most difficult thing to counter and obviously much depends on the attitude of the individual, but a lack of self-motivation does not indicate a lack of need.

(Holden, 1980).

I am quite often asked: 'What do you feel about having motor neurone disease?' The answer is, I try to lead as normal life as possible, and not think about my condition, or regret the things it prevents me from doing, which are not that many.

(Hawking, 1989).

The way in which individuals react to their illness depends largely upon their basic personality. MND, as an illness, is characterized by the various losses imposed upon the patient and family. It would be easy for them to 'tend towards an almost chronic state of depression' (Woodcock, 1985), but many find the inner strength to 'fight "the enemy" tooth and nail to the bitter end' (Pollard, 1984).

Some people are able to do this with the help of family and friends alone but many need the help of health professionals to explain facilities available, equipment to help them in their task and provide encouragement to aim for a better quality of life. This aspect of the care of people suffering from MND can be amongst the most rewarding to the health professionals as it requires use of all the skills learnt through training and beyond, and a willingness to learn from the people to whom help is offered.

CONCLUSION

This stage of care for people with MND can last for many months or years. There are many areas in which the health professionals can provide help and support on a practical as well as an emotional level.

'No matter how much I do, I always feel I should be doing more.' These words have been spoken repeatedly in relation to the care of people with MND. It important to evaluate the care and intervention offered to these families constantly and it should be adjusted accordingly. If there is any doubt a discussion with the patient and family will usually reveal any areas in which there is too much or too little help. During this stage more than any other it is true to say that while this disease may be incurable, it is not untreatable.

REFERENCES

Barney, J. (1993) Counselling Danny. *Reader's Digest*, July.

Bosma, J. F. and Brodie, D. R. (1969) Disability of the pharynx in amyotrophic lateral sclerosis as demonstrated by cineradiography. *Radiology*, **92**, 97–103.

Hawking, S. (1989) *A brief history of disability*, 6 April.

Henke, E. (1968) Motor neurone disease – a patient's view. *B.M.J.*, **2**, 765.

Hicks, F. and Corcoran, G. (1993) Should hospices offer respite admissions to patients with motor neurone disease? *Palliative Medicine*, **7**, 145–50.

Holden, T. (1980) Patiently speaking. *Nursing Times*, June 12, 1035–6.

Kaye, P. (1991) *Symptom Control in Hospice and Palliative Care* (3rd edn), Hospice Education Institute, Connecticut, USA.

Langton-Hewer, R. (1988) *Motor Neurone Disease: Rehabilitation of the Physically Disabled Adult*, Chapman & Hall, London.

Leik, N. and Davidson-Neilsen, M. (1987) *Healing Pain*, Tavistock/Routledge, London.

Maslow, A. (1968) *Towards a Psychology of Being* (2nd edn), Van Nostrand-Reinhold, New York.

Mearns, D. and Thorne, B. (1992) *Person Centred Counselling in Action*, Sage Publications, London.

Newrick, P. G. and Langton-Hewer, R. (1984) Motor neurone disease: can we do better? A study of 42 patients. *B.M.J.*, **289**, 539–42.

Norris, F. H., Smith, R. A. and Denys, E. H. (1985) Motor neurone disease: towards better care. *B.M.J.*, **291**, 259–62.

Oliver, D. (1988) Syringe drivers in palliative care: a review. *Palliative Medicine*, **2**, 21–6.

Oppenheimer, E. A. (1993) Decision-making in the respiratory care of amyotrophic lateral sclerosis: should home ventilation be used? *Palliative Medicine*, **7** (Suppl. 2), 49–64.

Park, R. H. R., Allison, M. C., Lang, J. *et al.* (1992) Randomized comparison of percutaneous endoscopic gatrostomy and nasogastric tube feeding in patients with persisting neurological dysphagia. *B.M.J.*, **304**, 1406–9.

Pollard, D. (1984) Personal view. *B.M.J.*, **288**, 481

Saunders, C., Walsh, T. D., and Smith, M. (1981) Hospice care in motor neurone disease, in *Hospice – The Living Idea*, (eds C. Saunders, D. H. Summers and N. Teller), Edward Arnold, London.

Stedeford, A. (1984) *Facing Death*, Heinemann Medical, Oxford.

Tatelbaum, J. (1981) *The Courage To Grieve*, Cedar Books, London.

Webb, C. (1985) *Sexuality, Nursing and Health*, John Wiley and Sons, Chichester.

Woodcock, J. D. V. (1985) Personal paper: motor neurone disease. *NZ Med.*, **98**, 1043–5.

FURTHER READING

Callanan, M. and Kelley, P. (1992) *Final Gifts*, Hodder and Stoughton, London.

Carus, R. (1980) Motor neurone disease: a demeaning illness. *B.M.J.*, February 16, 455–6.

Cochrane, G. M. (1987) *The Management of Motor Neurone Disease*, Churchill Livingstone, Edinburgh.

Gibb, M. (1989) Motor neuron disease: a patient's view. *Clin. Rehabil.*, **3**, 305–6.

Griffiths, G. (1982) Where there's hope there's life. *The Practitioner*, **226**, August, 1365–6.

Kubler-Ross, E. (1970) *On Death and Dying*, Tavistock, London.

MNDA. *Symptom Control in Motor Neurone Disease*, Motor Neurone Disease Association, Northampton.

Murray-Parkes, C. (1970) *Bereavement*, Penguin Books, Harmondsworth.

Speck, P. (1978) *Loss and Grief in Medicine*, Bailliere Tindall, London.

Wilson, B. (1982) Battling with motor neurone disease. *B.M.J.*, **284**, January 2, 34–5.

7

Terminal care

*You don't have to **do** anything. Being there is enough.*
(Jack Davies, 1993).

INTRODUCTION

Jack had been living with MND for three and a half years when the incident occurred that provoked this comment. He had recently been admitted to hospital with a severe chest infection which was responding to antibiotic treatment, and he had developed a very productive cough. The muscles in his chest wall were weak and his diaphragm, whilst comparatively strong, was unable to provide enough power to clear the secretions produced.

If he were not to exhaust himself completely, Jack needed the help of a physiotherapist to assist in clearing his chest but no one was available at the time. As an occupational therapist, I had used assisted coughing techniques in times of emergency and was asked to help.

Problem solving forms a significant part of the role of an occupational therapist and practical solutions can be comforting to patient and therapist alike. The progression of Jack's illness had reached a stage where few practical solutions were now needed. Jack's cough settled eventually and there was time to discuss the satisfaction experienced through practicality. After much thought, Jack made the observation which is quoted at the beginning of this chapter.

To suggest that there is nothing practical that can and should be done to help people in the terminal stage of MND would be misleading. As will be discussed during this chapter, people in this situation have many needs both physical and psychological.

Jack was talking about a different dimension to care in the terminal stage of his illness. He was referring to the courage and conviction needed by health professionals to remain involved in a person's care, even when they think that there is no useful function they can perform. He responded spiritually to a statement made from a physical standpoint.

Occupational therapy can be defined as 'mental or physical activity designed to assist recovery from disease or injury' (*Oxford Modern English Dictionary*, 1992). Working in the field of palliative medicine, recovery may take the form of resolution of pain, distress or unfinished business accumulated over many years. The activity may be talking, listening, creating, visiting new places or revisiting old ones.

Caring for people during the terminal phase of their illness is a privilege, as most people working in this area will relate. It is also time consuming and may be painful and sad but the rewards are immeasurable. The terminal stage of an illness is usually recognized as being the last few days or hours of life, when the person's physical condition has deteriorated to a state where it is no longer able to support life. Whilst this is true for people suffering from MND, the terminal phase can in some cases also involve the weeks prior to death.

The progression of this illness is such that it affects different muscles unpredictably. In some cases, the vital muscles of breathing or swallowing can be weakened to a state where it may be impossible to determine whether death is imminent or whether the person has some weeks left to live. For this reason, terminal care in this chapter will be expanded to cover this eventuality. Terminal care of the type offered to many people suffering from incurable cancer is also appropriate to people in the terminal state of MND.

Hospice philosophy travels well and the model can be used by health professionals working with different client groups. Palliative care can be used effectively during the progression of the illness and the application of terminal care techniques can reduce pain and anxiety at the end of life.

FACING DEATH

At the time of diagnosis, people with MND and their families are encouraged to concentrate on living and, whilst most are aware of the future, few dwell on the issues surrounding death. As the disease progresses and muscle control deteriorates, the reality of the illness is felt. It is not unusual for a patient or carer to say 'I knew this was going to happen but I didn't really understand what it would be like'.

In many ways, this can be a positive response. If the full implications were apparent from the onset of the illness, the patient and family would be unable to function through the early stages of the disease. The way in which a person faces death is usually characteristic of the way in which they live, but certain external factors experienced by most people with MND may be relevant.

Physical deterioration

'Look at that hand – it does not even feel as if it belongs to me and it seems to have a will of its own.' Frank was voicing his anxiety and disgust at the wasted muscles of his hand and the continual fasciculations he saw.

Physical deterioration is obvious to the patient and carer. The weakening muscles allow less movement and functional activity is gradually lost. In addition to this, muscle bulk may be lost which dramatically alters the patient's physical appearance. Attention to physical appearance is important despite the degree of deterioration experienced by the patient. It may not be possible to restore a person's original appearance but it will be possible to maximize his assets.

If physical changes in appearance are great, it is not unknown for the carer to have increasing difficulty relating to the patient. The person with whom she was familiar may have gradually changed into someone she does not recognize. This may form part of the separation process as both the patient and carer become aware that life expectancy is now short. The carer can become distressed if this is not understood, and the patient may feel rejected if he becomes aware of the carer's feelings towards him.

Making a will

Ideally, every adult should make a will; however, most people are reluctant to take this step unless they are encouraged to do so by external pressure. Making a will requires that people acknowledge their mortality and many feel it is morbid and 'might hasten the end'. People with MND are no exception. Through the earlier stages of the illness they concentrate on living and many may be reluctant to make a will at that stage.

Making a will can be a positive step. It enables patients to retain control over their life by ensuring that their wishes for the future will be followed. Even if the will is straightforward, it can reduce lengthy legal proceedings following the death of the patient.

Where the patient has children younger than the age of consent, consideration should be given to their future care and guardianship. Children's security can be threatened by the death of a parent, and they will need to know that their future is secure should the other parent die also.

Many large firms of solicitors offer the service of visiting the patient in his own home if travelling is difficult and have provision should the person be unable to write. In the case of a married couple, they recommend that both make their will together.

Physical dependence

When a person is diagnosed as having MND, he should be given the information he requires to begin to understand the illness with which he is living. Part of this information will involve discussion of the functions which may become affected and the functions which usually remain intact.

People with MND rarely feel unwell unless they are suffering from pain, discomfort or infection. This remains true throughout the illness often to within a few hours of death. It can be hard for a person to accept dependence on others when he feels well in himself.

Dislike of dependence may be expressed in many ways. Anger is common and may be expressed openly or with more subtlety. Acceptance of the true situation may be suspended, as with one young man who told his wife angrily that he was going to get up and walk across the room, despite his inability to bear weight.

Encouraging the patient and carer to understand the reason for these outbursts can help to reduce the power of the attack. Despite this, the carer may still feel that the outburst is a personal criticism of her or her ability to cope. At this time, the responsibility of care for the patient will probably have fallen to the main carer during the preceding months or years. Exhaustion can lead to the carer feeling that despite her efforts she cannot get anything right. In addition, she has no energy to try harder.

Time should be taken to explore the reasons for angry outbursts which are often precipitated by the carer attempting to respond to excessive demands from the patient. Even at this stage of the illness, the carer may need to delegate some of the tasks involved in caring for the patient. Admission of this need can seem like failure to the carer who may require support and reassurance to overcome emotions experienced.

Health professionals working in this situation will need to be aware of the pressures experienced by these people, and allow time for the patient and/or carer to voice their anxieties. Many carers are new to the task and may think that their feelings are irrational and wrong. A non-judgemental approach allows the carer to verbalize any worries.

Despite the severity of the disease and the physical constraints this places upon the patient, many wish to and are able to contribute to decision-making until the end of their life. If speech is poor, communicators can be used, and active participation should be encouraged for as long as the patient wishes.

Emotional dependence

Physical dependence may be accompanied by emotional dependence. Many people who become physically dependent as a result of MND feel anxious and frightened. Breathlessness, choking attacks or loss of muscle control may cause anxiety and some patients feel reassured by the presence of a trusted helper. Other patients are unable to verbalize their fears and the anxieties which result may show in the patient making unrealistic demands on the carer. Requests for frequent repositioning or toileting may carry a hidden request for companionship and reassurance.

This behaviour can be exhausting for the carer and can cause friction between the patient and carer, especially if the patient is unaware of his behaviour. Offers by friends and other members of the family to visit and spend time with the patient can reduce the pressure on the main carer. Carers from Crossroads care scheme or similar local agencies may be able to help if family and friends are unavailable.

This stage of the illness can be the most difficult for the carer. The patient usually requires total care during the day and, even if he is able to sleep at night (many find this difficult, despite sedation), he will probably require repositioning frequently. Acceptance of the inevitability of the illness can be hard to acknowledge for patient and carer alike as the following case study illustrates.

Steve had lived with MND for three years. He had been cared for by Mandy, his wife, at home during this time. His condition had deteriorated quickly at the onset and his chest muscles and diaphragm weakened swiftly threatening a poor prognosis.

In the early stages of the illness, Mandy was able to leave Steve on his own for periods of time whilst she went shopping or collected their children from school. Following a fall at home, Steve asked not to be left on his own when Mandy was out. Arrangements were made for a nurse to sit with Steve once a week to enable Mandy to go out. This arrangement worked initially, but Steve became anxious as he felt that the nurse would not understand his speech and know what he wanted.

He refused offers from friends and relatives to stay with him on the same grounds, which prevented Mandy from going out except for very short periods of time. Steve had reached a stage of emotional dependence on Mandy which paralysed Mandy's life as much as the MND was paralysing his own.

This situation continued for some months before Mandy reached a state of exhaustion. Steve was admitted to the local palliative care unit to enable Mandy to rest. He was extremely unhappy with this arrangement but had no other choice since Mandy was temporarily unable to care for him. On discharge, he was still reluctant for Mandy to accept any help at home, despite this experience.

This situation arose because Steve had become so weak that he was thought to have only a short time left to live. Mandy was reluctant to force the issue because his weakened condition suggested that he was in the terminal stage of the illness. Steve lived for eight months following this incident.

With the benefit of hindsight, Mandy realized that she should have insisted on provisions for respite care and help within the home earlier.

Arrangements for respite care and appropriate help at home, if addressed at an early stage in the illness, can prevent this type of dependence.

Emotional dependence can be reduced if the health professionals involved in patient care encourage the patient and carer to explore this potentially sensitive area and reach a resolution. Outside help in the form of sitters or companions needs to be established before speech becomes incoherent or mobility deteriorates severely.

Resolution of unfinished business

Throughout life, relationships are made and broken, altered, suspended and renewed. Whilst each person knows that life is finite, thought is rarely given to how or when that life will end. Diagnosis of an illness like MND can cause a person to evaluate life, and gives an opportunity to address some of the resentments, great or small, which may have occurred in the past.

During the progression of the illness the patient often has plenty of time to think and identify areas of concern, but may need help to work through thoughts and take the action required to bring about reconciliation. In many instances, forgiveness may not involve another person, but may necessitate permission to forgive oneself.

> Heavy, unresolved personal guilt or deep bitterness towards another seems to trap them (the patient) in their own agony, unable to 'let go' into death.
>
> *(Clark, 1990)*.

This was illustrated clearly by Jack, mentioned at the beginning of this chapter. The chest infection which resulted in his admission to hospital was severe and most of the staff on the ward were convinced that he was too weak to survive. Jack, however, had unfinished business which prevented him from letting go at that time.

During the weeks following his recovery from the infection, Jack remained in hospital since he needed total nursing care. He was a consummate communicator who enjoyed telling yarns and listening to other people's problems. He was reluctant to talk about himself, but gradually accepted the opportunity offered him to look back over his life.

He had led an interesting life, but like all of us had done things he regretted. His many friends and acquaintances thought highly of him, and whilst they had forgiven him, he had been unable to forgive himself. Time spent working through the feelings related to these incidents allowed self-forgiveness and three months later he died peacefully.

Most people who work with the terminally ill recognize the need to work through unresolved feelings. Ultimately the desire rests with the patient and family and whilst health professionals may see the need and indicate a willingness to help, not all patients will respond. Many people with MND regard their ability to retain control over their lives as vital and this should be respected here, as in other areas.

EUTHANASIA

This issue has been debated at length by many eminent people involved in the care of the dying, from both the moral and legal viewpoint. Saunders (1990), Lamerton (1985) and Hinton (1967) include sections addressing euthanasia in their works on care of people living with terminal illness. At this time, euthanasia is illegal in Great Britain, although the debate continues for and against its legalization. 'Exit' (originally the Euthanasia Society) and groups allied to its thinking argue the case for the introduction of voluntary euthanasia.

The hospice movement, along with many people who work with the terminally ill, strongly opposes the legalization of voluntary euthanasia. The effects of MND can be severely disabling towards the end of life and many people, on seeing someone with advanced MND for the first time, cannot imagine how a person would want to continue living under such conditions. In most instances people do, passionately.

Euthanasia can be defined as 'the bringing about of a gentle and easy death in the case of incurable and painful disease' (*Oxford Modern English Dictionary*, 1992). Most people facing terminal illness experience feelings of despair, but when given time to discuss these feelings further, find they are related to a specific problem. If this problem is addressed and where possible removed or reduced, life becomes more bearable again. Copperman (1983) writes 'I believe that suicide, actual or attempted, is comparatively rare, because for most people life is sweet, however distorted we as observers may consider their lives to have become'.

It would be unrealistic to expect that anyone living with an illness like MND would not experience periods of despair, but feelings of uselessness, dependence and sorrow can be reduced if opportunity is given to express them openly. A further example from Jack's case study illustrates this point.

Jack spent one afternoon talking about how much he hated the restrictions placed upon him by his illness. He said he felt that life was worthless since he had lost so much. He had been visited earlier by the ward doctor who had diagnosed a chest infection and had prescribed antibiotic treatment.

Further discussion centred on this infection, the proposed treatment, the likely outcome if the treatment was refused and his rights as a patient to accept or refuse any treatment offered. During this discussion Jack expressed anger and frustration at his present situation. Following this, talk reverted to ever-present ward gossip.

When offered the antibiotics by the nurse carrying out the drug round, Jack accepted the tablets. The reason for this, he said, was that he was not ready to give up yet.

'I want to die' expresses anguish that demands attentive and experienced listening. Once again, the team member must try to disentangle the reasons for this wish. It often arises when past treatment for distress has been inept and listening cursory.

(Saunders, 1990).

If a person felt that his medical team may take him at his word, opportunities for discussions of this kind would probably be reduced. Relatives have, on occasion, said of a patient 'He always said if it came to this (a catheter, maybe, or proposed move to residential care) that he would rather die'. In reality, when faced with the situation and given the support to think about it and discuss the options, the patient rarely chooses death as the solution – often to the surprise of his family.

Life is precious and a person who is terminally ill has the right to treatment to alleviate pain and suffering. Such treatment is aimed at improving the quality rather than the quantity of life left to a patient and, whilst on occasion a person may live for a few days or weeks longer through the administration of good symptom control, this is not the primary aim of the treatment.

NEEDS OF THE DYING PATIENT

To work in a team looking after a person with Motor Neurone Disease is often frustrating and exhausting. But to share with someone suffering from such a devastating disease is to see enormous courage.
(Betty O'Gorman and Tony O'Brien in Saunders, 1990).

As with birth, death is an intensely personal event. It will be a unique occasion for each person and family and will touch the health professionals involved in their care, often quite profoundly.

The needs of a person with MND will be similar to those of a patient dying of any other progressive terminal illness. These people have a right to physical and psychological support appropriate to their needs and the special problems experienced by this patient group are addressed in the following section.

Physical care

By the terminal phase of the illness, most people with MND are able to perform few if any tasks for themselves. Increased assistance from family, friends and care services will be required to reduce pressure on the main carer at this time.

Sleep

Sleep may be affected if the patient is unable to move around in bed. Medication in the form of night sedation may be inappropriate if insomnia is caused by discomfort and the patient may need repositioning frequently during the night. Carers can become exhausted and the use of night sitters may be considered. Arrangements can be made privately or through care management if insufficient private funds are available.

Sensation is retained throughout the course of the illness. Care should be taken over provision of pressure-relieving cushions and mattresses to ensure that the skin remains intact. Prevention in this instance can save a great deal of suffering for the patient and time for the district nurse. The occupational therapist and/or district nurse will be able to advise on suitable types of cushions and mattresses.

People suffering from advanced MND are usually thought to be at high risk from pressure sores. Assessment charts such as the Waterlow Scale determine the level of risk and are required by many health authorities before provision of pressure-relieving mattresses will be considered. Some pressure-relieving mattresses are expensive to buy but many may be rented for periods of time, a solution which may be more cost-effective. Discussion between the district nurse, her superior and the relevant health authority will be necessary if this course of action is considered.

Personal care

District nurses or social services carers can help with daily care – washing, dressing and toileting. If transfers cause problems, a hoist may be obtained after assessment by a community occupational therapist. The main consideration surrounding this issue is the suitability of the patient's home for its use; the patient's physical condition will also affect the choice of sling.

Manual handling of patients with advanced MND should be undertaken with great care. As the muscles become weaker, joints become less stable and rough or careless handling can cause severe pain and damage to the joints.

In many instances, particularly where patients have some spasm in their legs, a standing transfer may be suitable. If health authority or social services staff are involved in caring for the patient, certain safety criteria must also be met. Following the introduction of health service lifting policies in many areas of the country, a risk assessment may need to be carried out by the district nurse or physiotherapist to establish the safest manual handling procedure for both the patient and staff.

Many people with MND become frightened when lying in bed and feel in greater control when sitting up in a chair. Use of reclining armchairs or wheelchairs with elevating leg rests and pressure-relieving cushions can enable this to happen, even if the disease is well advanced and the patient is severely disabled. The occupational therapist should be able to advise in this area of care.

Mouth care

Special attention should be paid to mouth care. A normal diet contains foods of differing textures which help to keep the mouth clean. People with advanced MND often need mashed or liquidized food and, in some cases, parenteral feeding has been commenced which reduces the natural cleaning and scaling process.

Reduced resistance to infection caused by the weakened condition of the patient and/or poor oral hygiene can result in gum disease, treatable by antibiotics, or oral thrush which responds to anti-fungal medication such as nystatin. In severe or recurrent fungal infections, ketaconazole has been found to be effective.

Sucking an ice cube wrapped in gauze (held firmly by the carer) can moisten the mouth where swallowing is severely restricted and has been found to be soothing. Use of glycerine and lemon mouth swabs is discouraged as they have a drying effect on the mouth; a cotton wool swab dipped in a solution of bicarbonate of soda is preferable.

Swallowing

Severe swallowing problems resulting in excessive coughing and choking can be frightening for both patient and carer. Plenty of time should be allowed for each meal and quantities should be kept small to avoid exhaustion. Many people dislike their food liquidized and prefer to restrict themselves to food they can manage when prepared as near normally as possible.

It is said that a relaxed atmosphere aids swallowing under these conditions but at this stage of the illness, both patient and carer are often tired and this may be a difficult goal to achieve, even if desirable. Whoever helps the patient with the meal should feel confident in the ability to relieve a choking attack, if one occurs.

Helping someone to eat where swallowing is a problem can be fraught with difficulties. Preparing food for a loved one is a basic human instinct and, if the food is refused, the carer can feel that it is she, as well as the food, that is being rejected. General tiredness of the carer, weakness and total dependence of the patient can result in anger and frustration being expressed. Patients and carers usually need a great deal of support to help them through this phase of the illness.

Swallowing may become an increasing problem as the physical disabilities become more severe. Consideration of parenteral feeding by gastrostomy in the terminal phase of the disease would be contra-indicated, since it would be unlikely that the patient could survive the anaesthetic. If the patient were excessively hungry or thirsty a nasogastric tube may be considered, but careful thought on the part of the patient, carer and medical team should be given to whether this is appropriate. If the disease is well advanced, heroic procedures can be distressing to the patient and carer and use of a syringe driver (see Chapter 6) is usually considered if the patient is agitated.

In most instances of severe swallowing problems during the terminal phase of illness, hunger and thirst are felt mildly, if at all. Excess fluids can cause severe coughing and choking, but intravenous fluids are rarely necessary since a dry mouth can be relieved by offering small amounts of fluid, jelly, ice cream or crushed ice.

Toileting

Toileting can become an area of difficulty. MND does not affect sphincter control directly and a man will often prefer to use a urine bottle rather than transfer on and off the toilet. It may also be possible to fit a 'uridom' or similar device for night use or for trips away from the home, to reduce the anxiety of whether toilet facilities are accessible.

Female urine collection systems are not so successful. If the patient worries that she will not get the toilet in time, frequent transfers on and off the toilet will be needed to prevent accidents. In the later stage of the illness it may be necessary to consider an indwelling catheter to reduce exhaustion of the patient and carer from these continual transfers.

Where people are unable to stand unaided, problems may be encountered in adjusting clothing before and after use of the toilet. The patient may need to be dressed and undressed lying on a bed but in some cases, a recliner chair may be suitable.

Constipation, often caused by nutritional intake, weakness of the abdominal muscles, certain medication, e.g. opiates, and lowered physical activity, should be avoided by use of adequate laxatives. If transfers on and off the toilet or commode cause problems for the carer, it may be necessary to control the bowel action by use of suppositories. This can enable bowel actions to be timed to coincide with visits by the district nurse.

The importance of bowel regularity cannot be over-emphasized. Even if the patient is taking little in the way of nourishment, it is still important that his bowels act every three to four days, unless the patient is comatose. Chronic constipation can cause severe pain and distress to the patient and distress to the carer.

Symptom control

Control of unpleasant symptoms is vital at all times during the course of the disease and should be continued throughout the terminal stage, with alterations as necessary. Syringe drivers (subcutaneous infusion pumps) ensure that the patient receives the correct amount of medication to keep them symptom free if swallowing difficulties are experienced. As has been said, they can be used at any time during the illness and can be set up by the general practitioner and district nurse and can be monitored daily within the home.

Pain and symptom control should be monitored and continued as the patient becomes weaker, through to death. Local hospice home care teams can be approached for advice on suitable medication if necessary, and many hospices now have experience in symptom control specifically for this patient group.

Breathlessness and excess secretions may cause a problem at this time. Opiate medication, as has been said, can help to alleviate breathlessness as well as pain, and hyoscine hydrobromide can help to control excess secretions. Both of these preparations can be obtained in forms that can be used in a syringe driver. In some instances, chlorpromazine may also be added to relieve agitation, but this has a more sedative effect than midazolam which reduces anxiety and spasm with fewer side effects.

The circulatory system is not directly affected by MND. It has been found, however, that prolonged inactivity, particularly in formerly active people, can predispose them to deep vein thrombosis. If untreated, this may progress to a pulmonary embolus. Pains in the calf muscles and increased heat in that area can be symptoms of this condition, and suspicious leg pain should be assessed by a medical practitioner as soon as possible. Pains in the chest caused by weakening muscles or joints are usually felt as a dull ache, but any sharp or severe chest pains should be investigated promptly.

Control

People with MND usually wish to retain control over their lives, despite weakness and ill health. It is important that their wishes are regarded where possible. Communication, however basic, will allow the patient to make his wishes known. Where communication difficulties exist, assumptions may be made on the patient's behalf. These assumptions are usually based on how the carer or family think they would feel in the same situation, and are often at variance with the patient's wishes. However weak the patient becomes, it is important to acknowledge his wishes and take time to discuss alternative solutions where necessary.

Location of care

The Patient's Charter and an emphasis by the government on community care have encouraged more people to exercise their rights regarding health care. It therefore follows that, if they suffer from a terminal illness, they also wish to choose where they would prefer to receive treatment and ultimately die. Most people, given the choice, appear to prefer to die at home, but will usually require excellent home care services for this to be achieved.

At the time of diagnosis, many decisions are made by the patient and family regarding the future and how or where the patient will receive care. It is important that people have a plan for their lives but as time and the illness progress, plans may need to be modified. Admission to hospital may be necessary as the progression of the illness is unpredictable, adequate support services may not be available or the patient may need monitoring that cannot be provided at home.

Care at home

Caring for someone with MND at home can present many problems. Although it may be the wish of the patient to be cared for and die at home, this may not always be realistic. The physical and emotional demands this can place on the carer and the physical toll the illness takes on the patient may result in the patient being admitted to hospital or hospice for terminal care.

Many patients are now cared for at home until the final few days of life. Infection, possibly bronchopneumonia, or severe physical disability may require hospital admission for symptom control and this may constitute a compromise in the eyes of the patient and family.

Busy hospital wards are rarely ideal places in which to spend the final days or weeks of life. Hospice care, where available, is usually preferable, but if this is not possible, hospice staff are usually prepared to liaise with hospital ward staff (at their request) to ensure good palliative care procedures.

Where the patient has received day care within a hospice, he will already be familiar with the surroundings. If he needs to be admitted for terminal care, the patient and family will feel more comfortable as relationships with the staff have already been established.

During the progression of the illness, the carer may have found it impossible to care for the patient at home and this may have required admission to a nursing home. Over a period of time, the staff usually become adept in nursing the patient and prefer that he remains at the nursing home through the terminal stage of the illness if at all possible. Advice may be sought from home care teams or Macmillan nurses if problems of symptom control arise.

Patients and relatives often have distinct ideas about provision of care for the patient. It is important to adhere to these where at all possible; however, as time and the illness progress, flexibility may be needed if the patient is to obtain the best care in the place most appropriate to his needs.

Transfer to hospital or hospice

The move to hospital may be, at least partially, expected and may be accepted easily. In other cases, it may require a radical change in expectations on the part of the patient and family. The effects of this move may be felt on a physical and/or emotional level.

Physical considerations

If the patient and family are familiar with the hospital through previous admissions, they will probably know many of the staff who, in turn, will be aware of the special needs of the patient. Conversely, the patient and family may be unfamiliar with the environment, and the staff may have little experience in caring for people with MND and the requirements of this patient group. In this case, the staff will need help and guidance until they are familiar with the patient and his preferences.

Hospital staff usually welcome help and assistance from the family on matters of personal care. Health professionals who have been involved in the community can also help to reduce the stress of the transfer to hospital by showing hospital staff how procedures have been carried out at home. In addition, they can help by visiting and continuing their support of the patient and their family if at all possible.

The family should be encouraged to offer as much care as they feel able. They may wish to remain heavily involved in the personal care of the patient, for whom they may have cared for many months or years;

however, some carers prefer to leave nursing care to nursing staff so that they can concentrate on more personal aspects of caring for the patient.

The most important area where the family can help occurs when speech is affected. Hospital staff will need to be advised on the methods of communication used and, in many cases, shown how they work. This was demonstrated clearly when a patient had his pyjama top removed by cutting open the back, because the hospital staff were not shown the patient's preferred method of communication and he was unable to tell them how his wife usually performed the task.

Some patients feel vulnerable when removed from their home surroundings and may ask for a family member to stay with them at all times. The patient may experience difficulties making and sustaining relationships when he is weak and time is short, and may feel more secure with a friend or family member present.

It is unlikely that heroic measures will be needed towards the end of life, the main aim being the comfort of the patient. The family should be encouraged to remain with the patient throughout the final hours or days if they wish, and regular conversations with the staff regarding the patient's condition, even if this seems obvious to the staff, will enable the family to plan breaks as necessary.

Emotional considerations

Emotions surrounding an unplanned admission to hospital or hospice can be intense. At this stage in the illness, there may be worries as to whether the patient will return home following the admission, whether they will recover from this infection or illness or, if they do, whether the carer would be able to cope at home again. These worries may be expressed through the following emotions.

1. Guilt

'I don't know why but I feel so guilty.' These words were spoken by the wife of a patient with advanced MND recently admitted to a hospice for terminal care. The patient had been cared for at home by his wife and daughter for nearly three years at considerable physical and emotional cost to the family, and was now suffering from pneumonia. He needed a high level of nursing and medical care, impractical to carry out at home.

Despite this, the family felt guilty. Their expectations had not been met. They had hoped to remain as a family at home until the end and instead had to settle for remaining as a family in the hospice. Demands placed on the family by the needs of a person with MND are immense. No amount of care is adequate and there is always the feeling that more can be done. Guilt is the emotion through which this is expressed.

2. Relief

The progression of the illness can be variable and often, if the patient is admitted to hospital just prior to death, the carer may be exhausted and feels relieved that the burden of care and responsibility has been taken from her.

Guilt may follow if the carer feels she ought to have been able to cope with the patient at home and often results if the individual attempts to live up to another's expectations. These feelings may not be based in reality, particularly if the patient is seriously ill, but the carer may need much reassurance that she has taken the right course of action in the given situation.

3. Fear

Fear usually results from a lack of information, poor communication and increased uncertainty. The patient is usually aware that the reason for his admission to hospital is a deterioration in his condition but is rarely aware of the seriousness of the deterioration.

It will be necessary for either the general practitioner before admission or the hospital doctor following admission to offer an opportunity to the patient and family for discussion of the reasons for the proposed admission. Again, explanations usually involve confirming the thoughts of the patient and family, but this can often dispel many fears.

4. Anger

Anger can also be a result of failure to meet expectations. The patient may feel angry and let down that his wishes to remain at home have not been regarded. Expression of this type of anger by the patient can result in the carer feeling guilty.

The carer may express anger against the hospital or nurses for their inability to care for the patient in the way she or the patient would like. Anger of this type is often attributable to the carer projecting her negative feelings away from herself and the patient. It is important for staff working in this area to remember that these emotions are rarely personal. Where possible, time should be allowed for the patient and family to express and work through their feelings in a safe, non-judgemental environment.

Communication

Communication is a skill which can be learned. The heart of good communication lies in the ability to listen creatively, hear what is being said, and respond accordingly.

(Beresford, in Turner, Foster and Johnson, 1992).

Kubler-Ross (1970), Hinton (1967), Lamerton (1985), Saunders (1990), Buckman (1988) and Copperman (1983) include sections in their publications on communicating with people who are terminally ill and/or dying. The importance of communicating with people who are terminally ill about their illness and the effect it is having on them is now widely recognized. In practice, it is still an area where many health professionals need to gain more knowledge and experience.

Throughout this book, the importance of communicating at each stage of the illness has been emphasized. Through communication, the health professional, patient and family will have developed a good working relationship, and communication during the terminal stage of the illness will be seen as a natural progression of the relationship.

General principles of communication apply here.

1. Time

   Ensure there is enough time available on both sides before embarking on an in-depth discussion. It can be embarrassing for the health professional and painful for the patient if the interview has to be cut short at an important point through poor time planning. People with MND often experience difficulty with speech (which will be discussed later in this section), so conversation may be slow and laborious, but none the less important.

2. Place

   Privacy is essential. No one feels comfortable talking about their feelings in the middle of a busy ward or department, or if there are people walking in and out of the room.

3. Mood

   Check that the patient feels that he wants to talk at that moment. People with MND tire easily and are usually at their best earlier in the day.

4. Listen

   It is impossible to know how other people feel but it is possible, by using the technique of empathizing, to imagine how they may be feeling given the circumstances in which they find themselves. This requires the listener to give her full attention to what is being said by the patient, not think about what she may say in return. It is only then that the listener can begin to understand how the patient is feeling. Listening in this way also demonstrates to the patient that the listener really wants to hear what he has to say. Making time to listen to how someone is feeling can help to make their life bearable.

5. Individuality

   MND is an unpredictable illness and whilst there are some symptoms which affect many people with the illness, they will not all affect everyone. In addition, the attitude of the individual towards his illness will have a bearing on how he will cope with the different symptoms. One person may find losing his ability to drive a car intolerable whilst another will despair over his inability to feed himself.

Care should be taken not to prejudge the situation on the grounds that the health professional has 'seen this before'. It is important to listen to the individual tell his own story; only then will the health professional be effective in offering help to the individual.

6. Reflect

The patient needs short responses to enable them to continue and to reassure them that the health professional is still listening. Prompts, such as 'I see', 'Yes' or even just 'Mmm', can be enough. Repeating the last two or three words of the patient's last sentence or reflecting back briefly upon the situation so far can reinforce that the listener has understood what has been said. It is important to ask the patient to clarify important points if in any doubt, to avoid misunderstandings.

7. Silences

Silences in the conversation usually occur when the patient is reflecting on what has been said or is thinking about what to say next. They are natural breaks in conversation and usually if left, the patient will continue. If not, a clarifying question such as 'You were saying that the loss of mobility made you feel useless, can you tell me more about that?' will help, or a question relating to an area that was mentioned but not explored earlier in the conversation.

8. Emotion

Many people are alarmed by passionate expression of emotions. These are not, however, unusual when people talk about their feelings, particularly related to their life expectancy. Anger and sadness are frequent responses to significant changes in a person's expectations and it can be helpful for the patient to feel secure enough to express them. At these times, there is rarely a verbal answer, but the power of touch – holding the person's hand or putting an arm round his shoulders – can say far more than words.

9. Painful feelings

At times, listening to another person's emotions can be painful. For instance, listening to a young father explore his anguish and sadness at not being able to see his daughters grow up and marry can evoke feelings of sadness in the health professional. Normal emotional responses will be experienced by the health professional, and crying with the patient in such a situation is not unusual. This is usually thought to be acceptable, providing it does not paralyse the health professional's ability to function within the conversation. It also shows a depth of caring by the health professional which is appreciated by the patient.

Remaining with the patient in his distress is important, and acknowledging feelings of intense emotion at what is being said can show the patient that the listener is trying to understand.

10. Rescuing

MND is an unpleasant disease. Rarely, when discussing its emotional effects, is practical help appropriate and it may be tempting for the health professional to try to rescue the situation and 'make things better'. Most people with MND need, at times, to be able to express their distress and despair at what the illness is doing to them and, whilst they would want a cure were it available, are aware that this is not possible.

In this situation, health professionals may be left with the negative and painful feelings expressed by the patient, who usually feels a good deal better at the end of the interview. Most health professionals have their own support network or ways to resolve these emotions. It is important that health professionals consider their own welfare and allow time to deal with these emotions following the interview.

Counselling

Provision for counselling varies throughout the country. Most professional counselling has to be sought privately since few health authorities are able to fund counselling services. In recent years, however, some general practices have begun to employ part-time counsellors to work with patients who require this service.

Most counselling undertaken with this patient group is of an informal nature and usually falls to one of the health professionals involved in the care of the patient. A good working knowledge of the illness can help her gain insight into the emotions and issues that may be present for the patient.

Communication difficulties

A significant obstacle to counselling with this patient group is that most people with advanced MND experience dysarthria to some degree (Saunders, Walsh and Smith, 1981). At best, the voice may have less volume than normal, at worst, speech may be incoherent and communication aids will be needed (see Chapter 6).

Relationships

As the illness progresses into the terminal phase, there may come a stage where some health professionals within the team caring for the patient and family question whether they should remain involved. This usually occurs because they do not feel they have anything to offer professionally. The physiotherapist may feel that any exercises are tiring the patient, who may exhibit a reluctance to be bothered with exercises anyway, or the occupational therapist may feel that the family have all the equipment and adaptations they require.

As the patient reaches the terminal phase of the illness, fatigue and weakness can become severe. This, together with communication difficulties, often means that the patient genuinely does not have enough energy to initiate and sustain new relationships or recommence relationships with people they have not seen regularly.

The family need a high level of support if they are to continue to care for the patient through this stage of the illness. Short visits and regular telephone contact should be maintained by health professionals even if they do not feel they are able to offer much practical help. The emotional and psychological support that they provide is immeasurable.

> Doctors of today should not feel that because they cannot cure patients with ALS (MND) they cannot help them. They can indeed help them by their compassionate understanding and friendship.
>
> *(Quoted in Kaye, 1991).*

As the patient becomes weaker and less well, expression of physical affection can become more difficult for the family. It is, however, a time when the patient may need constant reassurance, and touch – holding a person's hand or putting an arm round their shoulders – becomes even more important.

Transferring the patient (from bed to chair or wheelchair) may be one of the few times that it is possible to hold or cuddle the patient. This observation has been made by patients and relatives alike.

Bob was a 60-year-old gentleman with MND, seriously ill with pneumonia. Shortly before he died, his daughter was talking about the activities she would miss with her father. The most significant was transferring her father into the car. 'It was the only time that Dad gave me a cuddle and I shall miss that terribly. He used to hold onto me until I had got him settled safely then give me a little squeeze before he let go.'

Honesty

Most people with MND will relate that they feel physically well – 'it's just that my arms and legs won't move as I want them to'. As they reach the terminal phase of the illness, this still holds true. To an outsider, patients may appear physically very weak indeed but they may still feel reasonably well in themselves.

As time and the disease progress, the patient or family will often have questions about the illness they wish to ask. This may result if they have felt unable to ask them earlier, or they may be questions relating to this phase of the illness. There are few answers but: 'If there are any useful generalizations they can only be that "telling" very often turns out to be "confirming", that denial can be a useful defence mechanism: that almost every patient swings between accepting and denying; and that the doctor is seldom if ever justified in telling a downright lie though he may often demonstrate consummate skill and compassion in the way he slowly infuses the truth to his patient' (Doyle, 1987).

Patients and families will usually choose who they wish to ask, what they wish to ask and when they wish to ask for information. This is an emotional time and the questions asked may not always be clear. It can be helpful for the health professional to clarify the question to avoid ambiguities. The question 'What shall I do now?' asked by the wife of a patient who had just died was answered 'You don't need to do anything just yet', only to be countered with 'I don't mean now – I mean how shall I manage without him!'

At some time during the terminal phase of the illness, it is likely that the patient or a family member will ask how long the patient has left to live. The patient or family are usually aware that it is not possible to give a direct answer and rarely expect one – they are often asking for confirmation that, having become so weak and disabled, the patient will not have to suffer for much longer. Most people who work with the terminally ill develop their own response when asked how long the patient will live. If this issue is explored with the patient, the answer usually lies in confirming his thoughts on the matter.

Talking about death and dying is not easy when a person is in good health; it is even more difficult when that person has only a short time to live. Questions are rarely asked directly, and require the skill of the health professional to listen to the underlying messages with sensitivity, and ascertain the information that the patient is really seeking.

Life is precious and in most instances the patient is reluctant to give up without a fight, however weak he has become. To an outsider, the quality of life appears to be poor and it may be inconceivable to the carers that the patient should be able to live under such conditions. As has been said, honesty is vital but should never be brutal. It is impossible to soften the information but if the health professional can show care and concern by employing sensitivity in handling the truth, the patient and family can be helped through this difficult stage.

Vulnerability

When people are unable to care for themselves they often experience feelings of vulnerability. Most people with MND come to rely upon one or two significant carers for their needs and the possibility of their loss can cause great anxiety. Constant reassurance of continued support may be needed from the carer.

This in turn can place added strain on the carer who feels indispensable, and may worry about their own mortality. Understanding and support will be required of the professional carers involved, and time may be needed to discuss this and possibly plan for alternative care should the carer be unable to continue.

LETTING GO

Most people with MND die as a result of respiratory failure (O'Brien, Kelly and Saunders, 1992): 'In this series, 113 patients died in the hospice. Of these, 45 (40%) deteriorated suddenly and died within 12 hours; 20 (18%) died within 24 hours; 27 (24%) within three days, and 19 (17%) within 7 days. Two patients (2%) lived for more than a week after sudden deterioration'.

Saunders, Walsh and Smith (1981) relate that death usually follows swift deterioration (about one week) and is often precipitated by bronchial infection. Dyspnoea and increased weakness may then be present, which can be relieved by the use of opiates. Benzodiazepines (diazepam or midazolam) or chlorpromazine may be used to relieve agitation and hyoscine may be added to alleviate excess salivation and terminal bronchial secretions. This medication can be given by intramuscular injection or via a syringe driver.

It is very rare that death results from a choking attack but if this occurs, administration of diazepam rectally (Stesolid ®), followed by an injection of diamorphine, chlorpromazine and hyoscine, will alleviate breathlessness and help to restore a normal breathing pattern (see also Chapter 6).

The days immediately preceding death can be a difficult time. The patient usually has a general feeling of unease but can rarely isolate the reason. The family are often concerned on behalf of the patient and themselves and they will usually require frequent visits from medical and nursing staff whether they are at home or in hospital. Regular monitoring of the patient's condition is essential.

Treatment of respiratory infections with antibiotics at this stage of the illness may help to control unpleasant symptoms but can rarely cure the infection. It is important to remember that, in most cases, the patient should be given the choice as to whether such treatment is started. Where antibiotic treatment has already been commenced, it will be necessary to talk with the patient and family if such medication is thought to be ineffective and discontinuation is being considered.

Discussion of issues relating to medication can be helpful to the patient and family, and where possible should be carried out whilst the patient has the strength to contribute to the discussion. Many people with MND are keen to retain control of their lives and the treatment they receive. The patient will need to be asked whether a discussion about the next stage of treatment would be welcome to him, or whether he is content for these decisions to be made on his behalf.

Physical care takes the form of good nursing practice. The patient should be turned every two hours unless this causes obvious distress. If anti-cholinergic medication is used, care should be taken that the bladder is emptied regularly or the patient my become agitated. If the patient has a problem passing urine, an indwelling catheter should be passed.

All procedures should be explained to the patient and relatives who, in many cases, wish to help with the care of the patient. At this time it is common for relatives to need guidance in what to do, and they will often ask what is expected of them. They may need permission to sit with the patient and hold his hand, since touch is very important at this time. It is generally thought that the sense of touch is one of the last senses to be lost.

Another question often asked at this time is 'Can he hear us?'. It is thought that people who are dying can still hear, at least some of the time (Kaye, 1991). This can be reassuring to the relatives who may have unfinished business to resolve, an aspect which may be of particular relevance if deterioration has been sudden.

Other questions relating to the patient's condition should be answered as honestly and with as much sensitivity as possible. Many relatives wish to be informed of significant changes in the patient's condition that may be noticed by medical or nursing staff, but may not be clear to the untrained eye.

Family members may wish to remain with the patient as much as possible. It may be necessary for them to be given permission to have a break to rest and allow someone else to stay with the patient, on the understanding that they will be called if the patient's condition deteriorates. Some people, however, may feel uncomfortable being with a person who is dying. If, after discussion of possible fears, they still feel unable to remain with the patient, they may need reassurance and permission to leave the task to another person.

Many people have not witnessed death at close hand before and may be frightened of what might happen. It can be helpful for the doctor or nurse to talk this through with the relatives and offer to stay with them and the patient or visit very frequently through the terminal stage of the illness.

If, immediately prior to death, sedative medication is required to control distressing symptoms such as pain or breathlessness, the patient may become very drowsy, even comatose, a state from which he may not recover. Explanation of this point to the relatives can help to emphasize to them the seriousness of the patient's condition.

Following the death of the patient, the relatives should be encouraged to stay with the body for as long as they wish, to say their goodbyes. Some people wish to help in laying out the body and their help should be accepted. The length of time the family wish to stay with the patient varies and it is important to be flexible in this matter.

CONCLUSION

Palliative medicine has become the major driving force behind the shift from terminal to palliative care. If terminal care is not to be consumed by the broader speciality of palliative care, then thought should be given to their clear separation rather than their merger.

(Biswas in Clark, 1993).

People with MND require good palliative care through the course of their disease, but as they enter the terminal stage of their illness they will also need good terminal care. Pain and anxiety can be reduced by medication, but fear, sadness and anger require an empathetic listener who is prepared to stay calm and discuss these emotions where necessary.

I really think I now know how Mary felt as she sat at the foot of the cross whilst Jesus was crucified.

(Eileen Freeland, 1992).

These words were spoken by the mother of a young man who died from MND. 'Being there' for Richard's family as he was dying was painful and sad, but they were helped by the knowledge that Richard was sleeping peacefully, surrounded by people who cared about him, and he appeared not to be suffering. Watching a person and the family cope with the terminal effects of this disease can be extremely distressing, but this should not affect the quality of support given to the family at this time, which is vitally important.

REFERENCES

Buckman, R. (1988) *I Don't Know What to Say*, Papermac, Basingstoke.

Clark, D. (1993) *The Future for Palliative Care*, Open University Press, Buckingham.

Clark, R. (1990) Forgiveness in the hospice setting. *Pall. Med.*, **4**, 305–10.

Copperman, H. (1983) *Dying at Home*, John Wiley and Son, Chichester.

Doyle, D. (1987) *Domiciliary Terminal Care*, Churchill Livingstone, Edinburgh.

Hinton, J. (1967) *Dying*, Penguin, Harmondsworth.

Kaye, P. (1991) *Symptom Control in Hospice and Palliative Care* (revised edn), Hospice Education Institute, Connecticut, USA.

Kubler-Ross, E. (1970) *On Death and Dying*, Tavistock Publications, London.

Lamerton, R. (1985) *Care of the Dying* (revised edn), Penguin Books, Harmondsworth.

O'Brien, T., Kelly, M. and Saunders, C. (1992) Motor neurone disease: a hospice perspective. *B.M.J.*, **304**, 471–3.

Saunders, C. (1990) *Hospice and Palliative Care*, Edward Arnold, London.

Saunders, C., Walsh, T. D. and Smith, M. (1981) Chapter 6 in *Hospice – the Living Idea*, (eds C. Saunders, D. H. Summers and N. Teller), Edward Arnold, London, p. 131.

Turner, A., Foster, M. and Johnson, S. (eds) (1992) *Occupational Therapy and Physical Dysfunction*, Churchill Livingstone, Edinburgh.

FURTHER READING

Frankl, V. (1992) *Man's Search for Meaning* (5th edn), Hodder and Stoughton, London.

8 | Bereavement

Well, is that it? Has he gone?
(Doris Davies, 1993).

INTRODUCTION

After living with MND for four years, Jack and his family had become used to the worry of chest infections; they made Jack feel unwell for a few days but in the past had responded to antibiotic treatment. This time, however, the infection was more severe and Jack's chest muscles were weaker.

Jack died very peacefully in hospital, Doris was with him as he had wished. She stayed a while to say goodbye then returned home. Once there, life felt unreal. How could someone so full of life as Jack just not be here any more? Doris had known he was unwell and would die soon – but not today. Death is so final, it seemed to her that there must be something beyond this life. Doris was experiencing the first numbing shock that follows the death of a loved one. This is the anaesthetic that helps the bereaved person to cope through the first few days following the death.

> The pain of grief is just as much part of life as the joy of love; it is, perhaps, the price we pay for love, the cost of commitment.
>
> *(Parkes, 1986)*.

Each person will experience loss at some stage in their lives and the ensuing grief. Loss and grief are felt in proportion to the strength of the attachment that has developed. The pain of grief is probably the most severe pain that a human being will suffer.

GRIEF

Grief can be defined as 'deep or intense sorrow or mourning'. Mourning is 'the expression of deep sorrow, esp. for a dead person, by wearing of solemn dress' (*Oxford Modern English Dictionary* 1992). The expression of sorrow varies widely between different cultures. The British culture, typified by the 'stiff upper lip', allows little time or space for the expression of grief and the bereaved person may feel isolated and unable to express true emotions.

In contrast, other cultures encourage the wearing of solemn dress and an open expression of emotions. Bereaved people are expected to weep, show sadness overtly and relinquish control of their lives for some days. During this time they are comforted and attended by their families and the surrounding community. It is not unusual for a year to be set as a time of mourning, and whilst grieving may not be completed in that time, it allows the bereaved person space to begin the readjustment.

Recognition, experience and resolution of grief are vital if the individual is to continue to live a productive life in the future. Unfortunately, many people still believe that eight weeks or so after a bereavement, most people should be back to normal, often denying them the opportunity to complete the grieving process successfully.

Human attachment

What for convenience I am terming attachment theory is a way of conceptualising the propensity of human beings to make strong affectional bonds to particular others and of explaining the many forms of emotional distress and personality disturbance, including anxiety, anger, depression, and emotional detachment, to which unwilling separation and loss give rise.

(Bowlby, 1979).

Many psychologists and psychiatrists have studied the development of personal attachments formed between individuals. One of the best known of these, John Bowlby, devoted much of his life to work on the importance of children's early attachment patterns, and the effects these have on the child's ability to form relationships throughout life.

Bowlby asserted that these attachments were necessary for a person to feel safe, secure and healthy, and that they were founded in the relationship that the child built up with its mother (or mother-substitute) during the first years of the child's life. Disturbances in this basic bonding were found by Bowlby (1969) to cause difficulties in later social relationships and could ultimately cause psychiatric illness.

Robertson and Robertson (1967–73, working with Bowlby) filmed and documented many young children in brief separation (of less than one month) from their mothers. During the 1950s, 1960s and early 1970s residential nurseries were used by many families, providing an opportunity to observe separation behaviour. The Robertsons were able to identify distinct patterns of behaviour exhibited by these children in response to the separation. Where the child was placed into unfamiliar surroundings without an individual attachment (mother) figure, the child appeared to go through patterns of behaviour very similar to those experienced by people in mourning.

> Grief is not a set of symptoms which start after a loss and then gradually fade away. It involves a succession of clinical pictures which blend into and replace one another.
>
> *(Parkes, 1986).*

Grief has a very important function. It is the process that allows a person to experience the pain of separation and loss and work towards breaking the emotional attachments that have grown up between that person and the deceased. When completed, the bereaved person should be able to reinvest in his or her own life without feelings of guilt towards the memory of the deceased.

Grief and MND

The grieving process beings when a person is told he has an illness from which he will not recover. At the time of diagnosis, the person with MND and the family grieve the loss of their future together. As time goes on, they will experience many losses. Loss of mobility, loss of independence, loss of role; the list is long.

The members of the multidisciplinary team will have worked with the family for many months, possibly years, and will have come to know them well. In many ways, some of the team will have been viewed as friends by the patient and family. Following the death of the patient, these members of the team will be in an invaluable position to offer help as the family embark on this new stage of their lives.

'The family are seen as "too involved", too easily hurt by each other's grief' (Parkes, 1986). The patient's family will, however, need to talk about their feelings and will probably want to ask questions about the final stage of the illness. The amount of help they will need as the weeks and months progress will vary, but contact at significant points – birthdays, anniversaries and festivals – will be greatly appreciated.

Experiencing grief

> All grief theorists agree that grief must be worked through – there is some sort of natural progression and blending of feelings which must be experienced if a healthy adjustment to loss is to be achieved.
>
> *(Gross, 1992).*

The person who is mourning can be seen to experience many feelings and emotional states. Many theorists have described stages within the process of grieving. Worden (1991) also identifies 'tasks of mourning' which need to be completed before grief can be resolved; these he sees as a practical way of working through grief. He recognizes that 'stages of grief' lead to the expectation that the person will pass from one stage to another in rigid fashion; tasks, however, suggest that people will address issues in their own way, in their own time. In any event, feelings come and go throughout the time of active grieving.

Worden's four tasks of mourning can be summarized:

- to accept the reality of the loss;
- to work through the pain of grief;
- to adjust to an environment in which the deceased is missing;
- to emotionally relocate the deceased and move on with life.

PHASES OF GRIEVING

As has been stated, stages of grief can seem rigid; however, for ease of description, some framework is needed. It has been found by Parkes (1986), Bowlby (1980) and others that some feelings are more likely to be experienced at certain times following a bereavement. This gives rise to the concept of phases, which are outlined in the following sections.

Phase 1 : shock

I knew that Barry was going to die yet I was not prepared for the shock I felt when it happened.

(Celia Stevenson-Cleaver, 1990).

Many people find this to be true and are surprised when it happens to them. The deterioration of a person with MND is usually quite clear to see, and the patient is usually very weak and ill when death occurs. In addition, during the illness, the patient has suffered periods of being unwell, from which he has recovered. The carer often feels that this *status quo* will continue, even if intellectually she knows this is impossible.

The way in which a person dies has an effect on the surviving relatives. A person may develop severe breathing difficulties and die within a few hours or may develop a chest infection which may linger for some days. In the case of the former, a higher degree of shock will usually be felt than in the latter where the relatives have more time to adjust to the knowledge that death is imminent.

Emotions experienced at the time of death and during the following few days enable the person to function, whilst emphasizing the reality of the situation. One way in which reality can be emphasized is in telling others about the death. This can seem a difficult task, but the opportunity to talk about the deceased elicits comforting words from the listener which, in turn, reinforces the truth of the situation to the bereaved person. Until the person realizes fully that the deceased has died and will not return, it will be impossible for that person to start to work through the grieving process.

Numbness

I felt so numb that I could not cry when Richard died.

(Eileen Freeland, 1992).

However a person dies, the survivors will often feel numb immediately after the person's death. This may cause feelings of anxiety or guilt, if others are able to express sadness at this time by crying – either reaction is normal. Numbness protects people from the full force of their feelings, which can be helpful in most cases. If it persists for more than a few days or weeks, denial has usually taken the place of numbness and the bereaved person may be led to feel they have resolved their grief too soon.

Alarm

It is not unusual for numbness to be interspersed with periods of panic. There may or may not be an identifiable reason for this. On occasion, the effort of performing day-to-day functions may cause alarm, at other times, thoughts of the impending funeral or the prospect of having to cope alone in the future will produce periods of panic.

Anger

Immediately following the death, anger is usually felt in sharp outbursts, but is rarely sustained. It may suddenly break through the numbness and may be irrational and uncontrollable. This can be a worrying experience for the bereaved or their supporters at the time, but again is quite normal. This said, some people have observed that angry outbursts enabled them to feel that they were still alive during the unreality they felt at other times immediately following the death.

Loss of concentration/memory

It is not unusual for the bereaved to forget people they have seen or events that have occurred immediately following the death of someone close. This may be a cause for alarm, particularly if it disrupts normal routine, and people may need reassurance that it is a normal reaction at this time.

Once the initial shock of bereavement has worn off, periods of poor concentration and memory loss may occur for some time during bereavement, particularly during periods of stress or at the time of anniversaries.

Disturbances of appetite

Loss of appetite is not unusual following bereavement and may be accompanied by a feeling of fullness in the stomach. It may persist for some weeks, resulting in marked weight loss. Conversely, over-eating may be experienced in an attempt to compensate for the loss.

Sleep disturbances

These may take the form of difficulty in getting to sleep or waking early. Vivid dreams may occur at this time and may persist for some time.

Causes of sleep disturbances may vary: some people may dislike or be afraid of sleeping alone; others may be frightened that if they sleep, they too might die. Hours of wakefulness may be times when the person relives recent experiences and memories of the past.

Sleep disturbances are normal following bereavement and usually resolve themselves. Medication may be necessary, however, if sleeplessness prevents a person functioning during the daytime. Where sleep disturbances persist, further investigation may be necessary, particularly if there is a possibility of clinical depression being present.

Pain

Pain is very closely associated with grief. This pain is usually thought to be emotional; however, early in bereavement it may also be experienced as physical pain. The bereaved person may experience pain in a specific area, such as headaches, or as a generalized pain throughout the body. In common with other physical pain, it usually responds to pain-killing medication.

The initial phase of the grieving process helps the bereaved person to begin to make the loss real, whilst the numbness acts as an emotional cushion between the person and the outside world. The week following Jack's death illustrates this point well.

The day following Jack's death, Doris observed 'I'm glad I organized Jack's funeral yesterday when I still felt numb, I don't think I could have done it today'. Numbness was still felt, but shafts of reality were beginning to emerge. The days between Jack's death and his funeral were filled with unfamiliar experiences, and Doris needed guidance to perform tasks that would normally have been done without thought.

Although Jack had been in hospital for some weeks prior to his death, Doris's sleep patterns were disturbed and her world seemed unreal and hazy. Eating became a chore and her resistance to infection lowered.

The support of family and friends helped Doris to make the arrangements necessary at this time. She arranged the funeral as she thought Jack would have wanted it, with special music as a celebration of his life. Whilst it was a time of intense sadness his death started to become a reality.

Phase 2 : working through the pain

Sometimes the feelings are so strong that I think I must be going mad.

I'm sure I should not have to keep going over and over it in my mind like I do.

I ought to be over it by now.

The concept of emotional pain differs from one individual to another. Grief is not predictable and an individual may experience pain in different ways, while mourning the loss of different people. The statements above were made by people in the process of working through the many components of the pain of grief. Some, or all, of the following emotions may be felt at this time. There is no set order and since 'Neither the sun or death can be looked at with a steady eye' (La Rochefoucauld, 1613–80, in Hinton, 1967), emotions come and go with varying degrees of severity throughout this phase of mourning.

Confusion

Grief is not a constant state – like the tide, it ebbs and flows. Periods of intense emotion are interspersed with periods of calm which, in themselves, can feel unnerving. Changes in lifestyle brought about by the death and the fluctuating emotions caused by grief can produce feelings of disorganization and confusion. Normal functioning may be disturbed and the mind may be preoccupied with thoughts of the deceased, particularly the aspects surrounding the final illness and death.

For the carer of a person who has died as the result of MND, the changes in lifestyle are immense. Throughout the progression of the illness, the patient will have required ever-increasing physical and emotional support. The carer may have not only lost her closest friend, but also her way of life. She is faced with picking up the threads of her former life, of which she may not have been part for two or three years, and this life will have moved on without her.

Weeping

As the numbness lifts, there will be times of intense sorrow. Weeping allows expression to feelings of sorrow and pain and may offer temporary relief, but for many people, tears may be sparse. Sadness may feel so intense that the person is reluctant to allow themselves to cry, for fear they will not be able to stop. Reassurance may be needed that weeping is not an embarrassment to those supporting the bereaved at this time.

Anger

He had had so many infections before and recovered that I felt really angry with him for dying this time. I know that's silly but it's how I feel.

Anger is felt to some degree by most people experiencing bereavement. It can seem irrational, but is thought to be linked to the frustration of being unable to prevent the death, and the act of searching for the deceased.

Expressing anger at the deceased can seem quite wrong to some people. Professional carers may receive this anger which may be expressed in negative comments about the help they managed or failed to give. It can be hard for the professional carer to realize that these comments are not personal at a time when they are also feeling sad at the loss of the patient.

Conversely, the anger may be internalized. This can be more dangerous for the person concerned as it can lead to depression and may ultimately lead to thoughts of suicide. If helpers suspect that this may be happening, the bereaved person should be encouraged to seek professional help and the general practitioner should be contacted.

Anger is a powerful emotion. People who experience the emotion personally, or supporters at whom the anger is expressed, can find the experience uncomfortable or frightening. Despite this, the bereaved person needs to be encouraged to express feelings of anger, and direct them appropriately.

Guilt

As can be seen from the statements at the beginning of this section, guilt can be a heavy component of grief. It is usually expressed by words such as 'ought', 'should', 'if only', and often occurs most strongly if the patient and carer have not been closely involved with decisions about their care.

Reality testing (Worden, 1991) can help to resolve feelings of guilt. Questions like 'How would you have felt if it had happened to you?' or 'If you could ask him, what would he say?' can be employed to discover whether the guilt feelings have a foundation in reality.

Exhaustion

I was trying to sort out his clothes and I found I could only take one or two things off the hanger, then I had to sit down for a rest. I found it hard to understand why I felt so tired.

Excessive tiredness is often experienced by people during bereavement, whether following a sudden death or a protracted illness. The carer of a person who has had MND will also experience the exhaustion caused by weeks or months of caring for a person who has been heavily dependent on her for physical and emotional needs.

Dreams

Sleep may be disturbed during bereavement and dreams may become powerful or unpleasant. Dreams are one of the ways in which a person experiences and works through emotions and, as such, may feature the deceased as if he was still alive. As has been said, sleep disturbances usually resolve themselves without intervention, but if normal daily functioning is severely disrupted a night sedative may be necessary to restore a normal sleep pattern.

Decision-making

During the weeks and months that the person is ill, the carer, at times, may think about the future. One of the common thoughts at this time relates to how and where the surviving family will live following the death of the patient. Moving house, within the locality or to a different area of the country, may be considered in an attempt to escape from painful memories of the illness.

In reality, making decisions following the death of someone close is difficult, if not impossible. Many people who have made major decisions too soon after the death relate that with hindsight, they should have waited until their lives were more settled. Life during this phase of bereavement can feel uncertain and will feel more secure if not disrupted further by unnecessary decision-making.

Depression

Freud believed that in grief, the world looks poor and empty while in depression, the person feels poor and empty.

(Worden, 1991).

It is thought that most people suffer depressive feelings at some time during the grieving process. The components of grief and depression are similar in many ways; however, as grief proceeds, the episodes of intense sadness usually become less intrusive and gradually resolve.

People who are grieving often feel intense, heavy sadness which affects their lives, but this is not necessarily clinical depression. It has been identified that people who are clinically depressed have often experienced a significant loss or losses in the past. It is, therefore, important that medical help be sought if it is thought that intense sadness has developed into clinical depression.

Restlessness and searching

Restlessness and searching for the person who has been lost are two powerful components of the grieving process. Whilst the bereaved person may know intellectually that the loved one will not return, she may still feel the need to try to find the person she has lost.

Feelings of loneliness may begin to replace those of restlessness and the need to search, as the bereaved person gradually realizes that the loved one will not return. As grieving progresses, the void left by the deceased gradually fills and the loneliness begins to lessen.

Mitigation

Over the months, periods of intense grief will be felt. Initially, one episode may feel almost inseparable from the next and cause severe pain and anxiety. At first, the episodes may be spontaneous but as time progresses they may be triggered by significant happenings such as anniversaries, a piece of music or a photograph. It is usual for the intense emotions of the first few weeks to give way to emotions of gradually lessening ferocity.

Parkes (1986) observes, 'The mitigation of the overwhelming emotion of grief by avoidance of the full reality of the loss is a necessary part of "distancing", of keeping the implications of disaster at a distance so that they can be dealt with little by little.'

Many people derive much comfort from imagined talks with the deceased or by feeling that he is still near. Others may hear a sound or catch a glimpse of the deceased which makes them feel that he is close. The pain of bereavement can be overwhelming, and these types of experience often feel comforting at a time when life feels bleak.

If the person is able to acknowledge the loss of the deceased and has gone some way towards working through feelings relating to the separation that this causes, they will gradually begin to readjust to the changes in their life.

Phase 3 : reorganization and resolution

During this phase, the bereaved person works towards adjusting to a life without the deceased. It becomes possible to acknowledge his importance and accept that he is no longer alive, but the bereaved person may now feel able to contemplate continuing with her own life. It is during this phase that the bereaved person is able to say goodbye to the deceased and, if grieving has been successful, will be able to remember him without undue sadness.

Gradual return of normal functioning

The bereaved person will still experience periods when grief is painful; however, she will also notice that there are times when she wants to think about herself and the future. Eating and sleeping patterns return gradually to normal and emotions seem a little more ordered.

At this time, the deceased may still be thought of a great deal but he is not the only focus of attention. There will be more time to think about activities outside the immediate family and the person's sphere of interest will begin to enlarge.

Memories

Memories are still powerful and whilst some may be painful, others will be reminders of happy times. Gradually it is possible to think and talk of the deceased in a positive manner.

Sudden profound sadness

As time goes by and the bereaved work to reorganize their lives, they may feel that mourning is complete. They may, therefore, be surprised by periods of sudden, seemingly isolated, emotions.

I have memories of an incident following the death of a close friend. A week before the first anniversary of his death I experienced two days of memory loss – I was unable to remember the contents of conversations that had taken place minutes earlier. I felt quite unnerved by this experience until I realized that it must have been related to the anniversary.

Readjustment takes many months and during this time it is usual for reactions such as sudden crying, memory loss or anger to occur. Tatelbaum

(1983) concludes: 'Although we feel much stronger, we may still be working through our grief as intensely as before, but in more subtle, less obvious ways'.

Breaking emotional ties

Part of the work of this phase entails the bereaved gradually being able to break their emotional ties with the deceased. This needs to happen in order that the bereaved can develop in the future. For some, this occurs spontaneously as the person reassesses her life and takes on new commitments. For others, it may be necessary to let go or say goodbye to the deceased consciously, so that they can reinvest in their own lives.

Forming new attachments

Asking when mourning is finished is like asking how high is up?

(Worden, 1991).

There are many different views on when or whether mourning is complete. In practice, it seems that mourning, to a degree, may continue throughout life. That said, if grief has been acknowledged and experienced, it is also possible for people to reinvest in life and form new attachments.

Setting a time for bereavement to be resolved is impossible. Many people seem to feel that they are coping better a year later. However, following the death of someone close, it is not unusual for two years or more to elapse before a person feels able to reinvest in life.

For many, resolution is measured by the ability of the bereaved to adapt to new roles in life, think of the deceased without guilt, sorrow or regret and begin to form new attachments. In this way, the deceased is never totally lost but has been moved aside, enabling the bereaved person to live and grow.

INCOMPLETE GRIEVING

Normal grief is painful but necessary and by working through the feelings that this entails, it is possible for the bereaved to resume her life. There may, however, be situations where mourning is not completed. The area of incomplete grieving or pathological grief is one which has been the focus of much work and research.

Facilities for grief counselling or psychotherapy, whether individually or in groups, vary between different areas of the country. General practitioners usually have information concerning facilities available in their area and are usually able to help.

Grief counselling and grief therapy

Many people cope with grief through the support of family and friends. Some may need a little more help in the form of grief counselling to resolve normal grief and yet others may need grief therapy to resolve pathological grief.

In this country, grief counselling is not readily available to all people who have been bereaved, although it is recognized that some people are more likely to need it than others. As a result, recognition of the need for help can become somewhat haphazard in practice.

Whilst it would be impossible to detail all aspects of pathological grief here, health professionals working with terminally ill patients and their relatives need to have some idea of the problems they may face. In addition, it may be helpful to be aware of signs to watch for that may indicate that all is not well.

Delayed grief

To many, the experience of loss and grieving is painful and can seem overwhelming. If the experience becomes too intense for the individual to bear, she may be unable to complete the grieving process.

Characteristics of delayed grief are that the person often experiences a reaction to the loss at the time of death, but may appear to have recovered more quickly than would seem appropriate to the significance of the loss. Loss, if not experienced fully at the time, will be repressed but not forgotten. In this way it passes into the unconscious, where it may not be remembered, but will cause problems with the functional ability of the individual. Inappropriate, intense emotions may then be triggered at a later date by another death or a loss of another kind.

The reasons for delaying grief can vary. The person may feel so overwhelmed by feelings that she cannot bear to experience them at the time, putting them on hold until later. This may happen if the person feels isolated and that they have no one to help them through the grief – grief can feel very lonely. Courage, to many, involves the bearing of sorrow or pain in silence and fortitude – indeed many people refer to crying as 'breaking down'. This discourages the bereaved from expressing emotions, which they then have to try to resolve within themselves. This can result in denial of the pain at the time in order that the person can continue to function.

Finally, grief may be delayed if people feel that they have to remain strong to allow others to grieve. Facing grief head on is not easy. It is a learned response to loss and separation and if there has been little experience of this in the past, the person will probably need the help of a counsellor to complete mourning.

Chronic grief

Normal grief progresses, albeit slowly, throughout the time of mourning. For some, the process ceases to progress; they have experienced and worked through their feelings but they are unable to resolve their grief.

In many cases, the person concerned begins to realize that her feelings seem to have continued for too long at a given level, but others may experience difficulty in differentiating between protracted and chronic grief. Buckman (1988) suggests that:

> If you're not making progress at all, and everything that hurt six months ago still hurts in the same way and **with the same intensity** and you are still going over the events of the last few days of your friend's life, then you are stuck, and you should seek professional help.

Through grief, it should be possible to experience emotions and come to some form of resolution. It is unlikely that the deceased would be forgotten and there may still be sadness attached to his being absent, but it should be possible to continue with life none the less.

It is not possible to work to an exact time, but two years after the loss of someone close it is usual that grief is less intense than it was immediately following the death and the bereaved have begun to reorganize their lives. After this length of time, some people may be close to resolving their grief. A person still experiencing an intense grief reaction and an inability to continue with life after this length of time would probably need help to bring the grief to resolution.

Life can feel very bleak and lonely during mourning and many people have periods of feeling that life has no meaning. This, however, is distinct from suicidal thoughts or threats. Anyone who, during mourning, expresses thoughts of taking their own life or attempts to do so should be taken seriously. Contact with the general practitioner should be made immediately and any concerns should be discussed with him or her.

People who become severely depressed during mourning may also be at risk of suicidal thoughts. This can lead to a dilemma, particularly if suicidal thoughts are suspected but not voiced. Again, if there is concern about the physical or psychological safety of a person, the general practitioner should be informed.

Any emotion taken to extreme can be worrying and disabling. Many emotions can be experienced in relation to grief but if the bereaved person feels overwhelmed, she may either push the feelings to one side, causing delayed grief, or the feelings may be expressed excessively. Anxiety is often felt as a component of grief. If it develops into panic attacks or phobic behaviour, the person may need professional help. Medication may be prescribed for treatment of insomnia or anxiety and may be helpful in moderation. Excessive use of drugs (or alcohol), however, may require professional help.

In general, grief counselling can help people who are experiencing uncomplicated grief but to whom it may be unfamiliar. Grief therapy may be needed when a person is experiencing pathological or complicated grief.

CHILDREN AND GRIEF

John Bowlby, through his work on attachment and separation, has shown that children younger than six months old form attachments. He found that the most significant person to a young child is the mother or mother-substitute and separation from the child's mother (or mother-substitute), even for a few days, can cause a grief reaction. As the child grows and develops, it forms further attachments with other members of the family.

MND is often referred to as a disease of late middle age but in recent years, more people in their twenties, thirties and forties are being diagnosed. Many of these people have families which include young children who will need to be considered during the progression of the illness, at the time of and after the death of the patient.

Children are very perceptive and are aware of changes in their environment, even if these changes are not fully understood. Involving children in discussions which explain these changes usually enables them to cope with the new situation. Where children have been involved throughout the course of the illness, they will have seen the deterioration in the condition of the patient. They will probably have asked questions and will have received the necessary reassurance.

During the terminal stage of the illness, children are often very aware of the seriousness of the patient's condition and may be reluctant to leave the house without reassurance that they will be contacted if any changes occur. That said, they may also be anxious about staying in the house in case they are there at the time of death. Few children have witnessed death and rarely know what to expect.

Children, like adults, need to say goodbye in their own way. This may take the form of being present at the time of death, seeing the body afterwards or attending the funeral. It is important that they are asked about their wishes in this matter and allowed to do what they feel able to cope with, rather than what the adults around them think they should do.

Children's reaction to death may be worrying to an adult. They may express anger at disruption of their routine, laugh or seem not to understand and go off to play. They may express sadness on being told, but children are unable to maintain sadness over a long period of time. Times of sadness may be interspersed with laughter and play.

It may be necessary to encourage children to express feelings in ways acceptable to them. Play, drawing pictures or telling stories may be used at different times with younger children, whilst older ones will welcome an opportunity to talk through their feelings with someone they trust.

When a close member of the family dies as a result of MND, all the members of that family, including the children, will have been involved through the progression of the illness and will experience grief. Children may need more encouragement and help to express grief than adults, but if treated with honesty and respect, usually resolve their grief with surprising maturity (see also Chapter 5).

PARTICULAR CONSIDERATIONS OF MND

MND is a chronic deteriorating condition but it is rarely possible to determine over how long it will last. In most cases, death will follow many months or years of progressive illness. In a few cases, breathing and swallowing are severely affected early in the course of the disease and death may come suddenly, possibly as soon as two or three months after diagnosis.

Most of the special considerations relate to people whose illness has spanned many months or years of illness. The relatives of those whose death follows only a short period of illness will obviously experience a different perspective.

Sudden death

At the time of diagnosis, most people are told that the condition is unpredictable and unrelenting. They feel shocked and numb and gradually the patient and carer begin to adapt their lives to the expectation that the carer will have to look after the patient as he gradually becomes weaker. This adaptation often takes many weeks and most people, at the time of diagnosis, are able to take the time that they need to adapt to the new situation.

In some cases, however, the disease progresses swiftly. The family, in addition to taking in the diagnosis, find themselves spending much of their time looking after the patient as he becomes more dependent. When death follows quickly, it takes on the form of sudden death to these families. The following case study illustrates this point.

Barbara was diagnosed as having MND in the early part of September when she was admitted to hospital, following a fall, with a fractured femur. She had been experiencing weakness prior to her admission and investigations confirmed a diagnosis of MND. Following treatment for her fracture, she was discharged home and was cared for by her husband Derek.

During the following weeks, Barbara became wheelchair dependent but was still able to feed herself. She needed help with transfers but her speech was largely unaffected. The main problem at this time centred around talking with the family, adapting to the diagnosis, and addressing feelings of anxiety related to her breathlessness.

By the beginning of December, Barbara's breathlessness was more severe and admission to hospital became necessary where she was given oxygen which seemed to ease the problem. Despite these measures, her breathing deteriorated very quickly and she died two days later, three months after the initial diagnosis.

Derek and his family felt shocked at the speed of the deterioration which led to Barbara's death. There were many issues unresolved, the family had time to say goodbye immediately before Barbara died, but there were other matters they would have liked to have talked about, but were denied the opportunity.

The sudden death of the patient will have a bearing on how the family cope with their bereavement. If possible, bereavement support should be offered to these families during the first few months, as a standard procedure.

The healthcare team may also experience difficult emotions in these circumstances. There may be guilt attached to feelings of relief that the person was spared a long and disabling illness or that more help could have been offered to the family if the health professionals had been aware of the severity of the disease.

Anticipatory grief

Many deaths occur with some forewarning and it is during this period of anticipation that the potential survivor begins the task of mourning and begins to experience the various responses to grief.

(Worden, 1991).

Anticipatory grieving is the term given to grief that is experienced by the surviving relatives before the death of the patient. Parkes (1986) identified that where death occurred following a period of deteriorating illness, the survivors coped better with bereavement than those who experienced the sudden death of a loved one.

Through the progression of the disease, it becomes evident to the patient and carer that the patient will not survive the illness. This helps to reinforce the initial stage of grieving, i.e. making the death real. It is the time at which they begin mourning the loss of a joint future and the carer realizes that he or she will have to build a new life alone, after the death of the patient. Times of reality will be interspersed with times of denial, when the carer cannot believe that death will happen.

The carer can become worried by thoughts of her life continuing after the death of the patient and may need reassurance that she is not wishing the patient to die prematurely. She may feel many of the emotions of grieving usually associated with bereavement before the death of the patient, and whilst these can help her come to terms with the probable future, they will not replace bereavement after the death of the patient.

Anticipatory grieving is normal but problems may occur if the patient lives beyond the time expected. The following two brief case studies illustrate this point.

Steve's condition deteriorated quickly during the first year following diagnosis, and he soon needed help with most activities of daily living, transfers and mobility. The basal expansion of his lungs was poor and it seemed that he may not have long to live. His wife, Mandy, was aware of his weakened condition and had discussed the possibility that death was near with health professionals involved with Steve's care. Steve coped with his illness by denying its existence and refused to discuss the severity of his condition.

Over the following two years, deterioration of Steve's physical condition continued at a much slower speed. Mandy and their three daughters were fully involved in Steve's care and talked about Steve's impending death and their future together. A time came some months before Steve's death when their anticipatory grieving was complete.

As the weeks progressed, Mandy related that she knew intellectually that Steve was becoming less well but could not believe that he would ever die. She experienced periods of guilt when she felt she had wished him dead and needed a high level of reassurance that this was not the case.

Conversely, the carer may complete their anticipatory grieving early and withdraw from the patient before their death.

John spent the last few months of his life in the local hospice. His wife had visited regularly and taken an active part in John's care, but the staff on the unit expressed their concern when she began visiting less frequently and became distant. She also took a much less active part in John's care. During the months that John was ill, his wife had completed her anticipatory grieving but, unlike Mandy, was unable to continue to care for her husband.

Anticipatory grieving is normal and can help to prepare a person for life ahead. It should not, however, be thought that because a person has experienced this type of grief reaction she will not grieve after the death of the patient.

Shock

Many people are unprepared for the shock and intensity of emotion they feel after the death of a person from MND. As has been discussed above, there is usually plenty of opportunity to think and talk about the future. However well prepared people may think they are, they will still experience all the feelings associated with bereavement, but may work through them in a shorter time than if the patient had died suddenly.

Isolation

People with MND become gradually more dependent on their carers as the illness progresses. At the time that the patient dies, it is not unusual for the carer to be providing round-the-clock care. The patient and carer are usually receiving visits from many members of the healthcare team and have little time to themselves.

Once the initial shock of the death has worn off, the carer often discovers that she has far more time available to her than she has been used to over recent months, and can then feel isolated. It can be tempting to over-compensate and fill this void with activities in an attempt to mitigate the pain of grief.

The carer is usually extremely tired, often to the point of exhaustion, and needs time to recover her mental and physical energy. At this time, the carer needs to be encouraged to work through her grief before looking to reorganize her life and take on new commitments.

HELP FOR THE BEREAVED

Grief counselling and grief therapy are formal methods of helping people who have been bereaved. Some people, however, require less intensive support. The following are suggestions that any member of the healthcare team can consider offering to the carer following the death of the patient.

Friendship

Throughout the time that the patient has been unwell, the members of the healthcare team will have been involved with providing care for the family. Over this time it is likely that some members will have developed close relationships with the family which can be carried through into bereavement.

Talking about feelings is rarely easy, particularly following the death of someone close. Many people have difficulty accepting loss and death and it can be hard to hear and cope with the feelings that this will inevitably evoke, especially within the family group.

Friendship, and a willingness to listen to a person's grief at this time is the most valuable gift possible. It is not necessary to 'know what to say' as there is often nothing that can be said to improve the situation. The essential message here is to acknowledge feelings present at the time, and not be afraid to talk about the deceased if this is what the person wishes to do. Sharing memories can provide much comfort at this time.

Caring for someone with MND can be physically and emotionally exhausting and, whatever happens, the family will usually welcome the opportunity to discuss the previous weeks or months. They need reassurance that they did everything humanly possible to meet the patient's needs, and may need to talk through events leading up to and surrounding the death of the patient, whether they were present or not.

Practical help

Following the death of someone from MND, there is often much to be done and most people have the support of family and friends to arrange the funeral. It is necessary to check that someone is performing this role; if not, an offer of help in this area will be appreciated by the carer, whether or not it is accepted.

Checking benefit entitlements at this time may seem callous, but some benefits change following the death of a close relative. The carer may need help coping with the inevitable forms that require completion.

It will be necessary to find out from the family how they wish to deal with returning equipment. Some people need the equipment removed as soon as possible – they find that its presence provides a constant reminder of illness. Others will need a few days to adjust to the new situation before dealing with equipment. If asked, most people are willing to discuss their wishes on this matter.

Self-help groups

Many hospices or home care teams offer bereavement support in the form of support groups or individual counselling, but many people with MND do not have links to a hospice. CRUSE or The Society of Compassionate Friends are both national self-help organizations, with branches in most areas of Great Britain. In addition, there may be local self-help groups set up to meet the needs of bereaved people within a specific locality.

Many people with MND and their families receive support from the local branches of the Motor Neurone Disease Association. During the patient's lifetime, the family may have had contact with a volunteer visitor who will usually continue support into bereavement. In addition, branch meetings provide a focus for fundraising to improve patient care or research into the illness. Many people who have received help from their local branch wish to offer help in return, as they begin to recover from their loss.

Parkes and Worden recognize the potential for volunteers working in this area of care. 'Busy doctors and social workers often lack the time to become good at bereavement counselling, whereas volunteers who choose to learn the necessary skills of this field of care soon achieve a high standard' (Parkes, 1986). People who have themselves experienced loss and resolved their own grief can, with training, offer much to those now experiencing loss.

SELF-CARE OF HEALTH PROFESSIONALS

Your pain is the breaking of the shell that encloses your understanding.
(Gibran, 1926).

Bowlby (1969) concludes that 'The loss of a loved person is one of the most intensely painful experiences any human being can suffer, and not only is it painful to experience, but also painful to witness, if only because we're impotent to help'.

Working with people who have MND stretches the physical and emotional resources of the health professional to the limit. The loss of a patient with whom the health professional has worked over many months or years will be felt deeply. Some of the most painful areas may not become apparent until after the patient has died. Working to resolve these problems can realize the truth in Gibran's words.

Worden (1991) considers the following issues in regard to grief counsellors. Many of the issues that are raised are equally applicable to those caring for people with MND and their families, throughout their illness and into bereavement.

Care for the carers

When faced with grief from a family, the healthcare professional may become aware of some issues that are significant to her. There may be losses that she has suffered in the past that were not adequately resolved. Helping a family with their grief may bring this into the foreground and most people would find it difficult, if not impossible, to continue to help without addressing their own problem first.

Facing grief with another person may also make the healthcare professional aware of losses she may fear herself. Helping a person who is grieving the loss of a child will be extremely difficult for the healthcare professional who finds this area difficult to come to terms with herself.

Finally, there may be unfinished business surrounding the healthcare professional's feelings associated with her own mortality. If this area or either of the others causes problems to the healthcare professional, she will need to resolve them, with help if necessary, before she can continue in this type of work.

Much is said but little seems to have been resolved regarding stress management and 'burnout' in relation to healthcare professionals. Working with people who are seriously ill causes stress, whether the condition is terminal or not. Support from within the team of people looking after the patient and family can be a great source of help. Worden (1991) has identified three areas which would seem to be fundamental to the continued health and well-being of people working in this area of care.

1. Identify personal limitations

Every healthcare professional has a limit to the number of patients with whom she can work at any one time. This number can be quite high if the amount of involvement with each patient is low or the relationship superficial. Where the healthcare professional is working at any depth with a patient and family, the number with whom she can work at that level is much lower.

It would be impossible to set a limit for the number of cases requiring a high level of involvement that any worker can take on, as each person is an individual. It is, however, necessary that the healthcare professional looks at this consciously and learns to recognize her own limitations.

2. Active grieving

Where a healthcare professional has been working closely with a family, she will experience grief following the death of the patient. This need not paralyse her abilities to help further, but it will be necessary that she acknowledges her own grief within the situation.

Coping with grief is an individual issue, but many people find that taking time out to attend the funeral is a helpful starting point. Following this, it will be necessary to allow time to experience the grief reaction that will inevitably follow.

3. Asking for and accepting help

Health professionals are notoriously bad at recognizing their own needs and asking for help. If she is required to work with severely disabled or terminally ill patients, it will be necessary that the health professional addresses this issue.

Once the need has been recognized, the healthcare professional will need to identify her support network, whom she can ask for help. This network may already exist naturally, as with the multidisciplinary team within a unit or within the community. If it does not, it will be necessary for her to organize supervision or the like through her line manager.

Experience in the area of palliative care can enable the healthcare professional to offer help in a situation where many who lack such experience flounder. This work is not without its difficulties. Healthcare professionals have needs which may have to be temporarily suspended in a crisis, but will have to be attended to as soon as possible, once the crisis is resolved. Emotions that are suppressed repeatedly will require resolution at a later date.

CONCLUSION

In order to help people through bereavement it is necessary to understand the various stages through which they will pass. In addition, it can be helpful to be able to recognize some areas that may indicate a problem, and areas that may create specific problems to the families of people who have died from MND.

Members of a team of healthcare professionals looking after a person with MND and the family will need support throughout the experience, continuing into bereavement. Self-care is an area that is often neglected but, ultimately, it is the responsibility of each team member to maintain their own physical and emotional health.

The care of people with MND and their families involves witnessing much sadness, which continues into bereavement. As the family gradually work through the process of grieving, much pleasure can be experienced through contributing to their recovery and watching them gradually learn to live again.

REFERENCES

Bowlby, J. (1969) *Attachment and Loss (Vol. 1 – Attachment)* (reprinted 1991), Penguin, Harmondsworth.

Bowlby, J. (1979) *The Making and Breaking of Affectional Bonds* (reprinted 1993), Routledge, London.

Bowlby, J. (1980) *Attachment and Loss (Vol. 3 – Loss)* (reprinted 1991), Penguin, Harmondsworth.

Buckman, R. (1988) *I Don't Know What to Say*, Papermac, Basingstoke.

Gibran, K. (1926) *The Prophet* (republished 1991), Pan Books, London.

Gross, R. (1992) *Psychology* (2nd edn), Hodder and Stoughton, London.

Hinton, J. (1967) *Dying*, Penguin, Harmondsworth.

Parkes, C. M. (1986) *Bereavement*, Penguin, Harmondsworth.

Robertson, J. and Robertson, J. (1967–73) *Young Children in Brief Separation* (film series), Tavistock Institute of Human Relations, London (films available from Concord Films Council, Ipswich, Suffolk).

Tatelbaum, J. (1983) *The Courage to Grieve*, Cedar Books, London.

Worden, J. W. (1991) *Grief Counselling and Grief Therapy* (2nd edn), Routledge, London.

FURTHER READING

Bowlby, J. (1973) *Attachment and Loss* (*Vol. 2 – Separation*) (reprinted 1991), Penguin, Harmondsworth.

Kay, P. (1991) *Symptom Control in Hospice and Palliative Medicine*, Hospice Education Institute, Connecticut, USA.

Lamerton, R. (1980) *Care of the Dying*, Penguin, Harmondsworth.

Leick, N. and Davidson-Neilsen, M. (1991) *Healing Pain*, Routledge, London.

Pincus, L. (1976) *Death in the Family*, Faber & Faber, London.

Staudacher, C. (1987) *Beyond Grief*, Souvenir Press (A & E) Ltd, London.

PART FOUR

Appendices

The next ten years are going to be crucial if we are going to conquer Motor Neurone Disease once and for all.

(Jamie Niven in MNDA, 1992/3).

This section contains information on practical help that is available to people with MND and their families: the work of the Motor Neurone Disease Association; names and addresses of helpful agencies; and examples of equipment that can improve independence for people with MND and their families.

Research continues throughout the world towards finding the cause of motor neurone disease, a treatment to slow the progression of the illness and eventually a cure. In the meantime, patients and their families need as much practical help as they see necessary to cope with the effects of this illness. If, as seems probable, a treatment is found that slows the progression of the illness, good management practices will be more important than ever.

Appendix A: The Motor Neurone Disease Association, UK

Motor neurone disease (MND) was described as a degenerative disease of the nervous system by Sir Charles Bell in 1830. Jean-Martin Charcot gave the first definitive description in 1865 and he was also the first person to use the name amyotrophic lateral sclerosis. Lord Brain, in 1961, suggested that the term motor neurone disease be used to describe the condition after it was found to have different subdivisions (Tew, 1991).

Despite knowing about the existence of MND for over 100 years, the Motor Neurone Disease Association (MNDA) was not formed in the UK until 1979, when three local groups which had been started joined together as a 'voluntary body with charitable status'. The overall aim was to bring together people with the illness, carers and professionals who were involved in the care of people with MND.

Peter Cardy, Director of MNDA, began a talk at the 1990 Conference of MNDA's Research Grantees thus: 'Most of our researchers know that the MNDA is unusual among medical charities – it embraces twin priorities of research and care rather than one or the other like most charities in the neuro-degenerative field'. These twin aims place considerable strain on the financial and managerial resources of the association and it is probably not an ideal way to run a charity.

Unfortunately, MND also places considerable strain on people with the illness, carers and healthcare professionals involved in providing a service. Research is undoubtedly necessary if a cure for the condition is to be found. Patient care services are equally necessary to enable the patients and their families to enjoy a reasonable quality of life.

MEDICAL RESEARCH

Research funded by the MNDA focuses on various aspects of the illness, both medical and clinical. Population studies help to determine whether environmental factors could be implicated. These can show where clusters of people with MND occur. Various studies are underway to determine whether environmental toxins, either artificial or natural, could cause MND.

It is also thought, following research, that certain substances may slow down the rate of deterioration in MND. The results of clinical trials using branched chain amino acids and more recent trials of riluzole (an anti-glutimate drug) will hopefully provide useful information.

Perhaps the most significant findings to date are those in the field of genetics. In March 1993, an international team of scientists identified a gene on chromosome 21 that is believed to be responsible for the familial type of MND. Further research is being carried out to discover if this could provide clues to the causes of the more common sporadic form of the disease.

MND is an illness that is found in most countries in the world. Research is being carried out in many of these countries and, in order to derive the most benefit from the different areas of research, the International Alliance of ALS/MND Associations has been launched. Its aim is to co-ordinate research and raise global awareness of the condition in medical circles. It is hoped that this co-operation between the nations of the world will help to accelerate progress in the field of medical research.

APPLIED RESEARCH

Whilst medical research is concerned with searching for a cause and cure for MND, applied research aims to develop equipment that will improve the quality of life for people living with the illness. Most of the work has been carried out at the Brunel Institute of Bioengineering, by a team headed by Professor Heinz Wolff. An autosip drinking aid, a portable bidet and advances in powered mobile arm supports have helped to increase independence for people with limited mobility.

Other areas of applied research include a project to identify better ways of caring for people with MND and their families at the time of diagnosis and how the use of a keyworker can improve care for people with MND through the progression of the disease.

CARE SERVICES

These cover all aspects of work by the MNDA to improve a patient's quality of life. They address many different areas that may concern a person with MND and the family, complementing the existing statutory services.

Statutory services should be provided for all people in the UK who are medically unwell, as set out in the Patient's Charter of April 1993. Unfortunately, the availability of these services may vary across the country. The MNDA works with healthcare professionals and statutory providers of care to ensure that people with MND receive care appropriate to their needs.

The MNDA is able to help financially in some circumstances to fund special pieces of equipment. People with MND face an ever-changing situation and when help is needed a prolonged wait can cause much distress.

Regional care advisors are employed by the MNDA to support and educate healthcare professionals working to provide patient care. They are also a vital link between the local branches in their area and the national office.

MND affects each person in a slightly different way, but many of the problems faced by these people have similarities. Getting up from a chair, sitting up in bed and problems with communication are a few of the situations common to many people with this illness. The equipment loan service aims to stock items such as electric riser/recliner armchairs, electric bed elevators and communication aids which are useful to people with MND but are not readily available through statutory loan services.

The most recent addition to the care service has been the MND helpline. Volunteers man the phones from 9 a.m. to 10 p.m. each weekday and it is hoped to extend the service to weekends in the future. The helpline provides a point of contact for people with MND and their families, who can obtain information about the illness and talk to someone who has some knowledge of MND.

Information leaflets are published by the MNDA and can be obtained from the national office by patients, carers and healthcare professionals on request. Factsheets on different aspects of management such as suggestions for clothing or different seating are also being developed, as is the service aimed to help children (particularly between seven and twelve years of age) whose mother, father or a close relative has MND.

MNDA co-ordinates many services for patient care from their national office located in Northampton and whilst this is centrally placed, it is still too far for many people to reach. More accessible are the 91 local branches of the MNDA made up of patients, carers and supporters who give their time voluntarily to support patients and their families, raise funds for equipment and research and raise public awareness of MND within their locality.

Each branch is run by a chairman, secretary and committee of elected members and most branches organize informal meetings and fundraising events, and provide a local point of contact for those interested in helping. Volunteer visitors, drawn from the local groups, are trained to visit and support people with MND and their families and are usually able to provide practical help and suggestions.

Over the last ten years there has been a steady improvement in care for people with MND and their families and this is largely due to the continued work of the MNDA. As the association continues to grow in experience and influence, it is hoped that the ultimate goal – a cure for MND – will not be too far in the future.

REFERENCES

MNDA (1992/3) *Annual Review: the Dawn of Hope*, Motor Neurone Disease Association, Northampton.

Tew, J. (1991) *The Plain Man's Guide to Susceptibility & Genes in MND/ALS*, MNDA, Northampton.

FURTHER READING

Cardy, P. (1993) Research and the association: an era for partnership. *Pall. Med.*, **7** (Suppl. 2), 3–9.

Cochrane, G. (1987) *The Management of Motor Neurone Disease*, Churchill Livingstone, Edinburgh.

MNDA Leaflet 1 *Motor Neurone Disease: An Introduction*, MNDA, Northampton.

MNDA Leaflet 5 *Motor Neurone Disease: Why Join Your Local Branch?*, MNDA, Northampton.

Appendix B: Equipment and suppliers

Motor neurone disease affects many of the muscles in the body causing people to lose mobility and independence in many areas of their lives. The information contained in the following section is not definitive but suggests some equipment that is available to help improve independence and quality of life. New equipment and models of existing equipment are being developed all the time and more people now have direct access to this equipment through a growing number of retail outlets and catalogue shops.

It is always advisable for the patient and family to check with an occupational therapist, physiotherapist or speech and language therapist before purchasing expensive equipment. This will ensure that the best item for that individual is purchased and that it would not be possible to borrow it instead, so saving the cost of purchase.

The MNDA national office will loan riser/recliner armchairs, Marcon bed elevators, portable suction machines and lightwriters (subject to availability) to people with MND, following an assessment by a healthcare professional. This service does not replace local loan systems, but can be used if waiting time for such equipment is lengthy.

EQUIPMENT

Mobility

Walking sticks   Standard aluminium adjustable
                              Cooper 'Fischer' moulded grip
Walking frames   Lightweight adjustable height
                              Lightweight wheeled adjustable height

	Folding wheeled frame
	Walk and sit frame
Wheelchairs	Manual
	Electric
Splints (available	Footdrop (Hartshill)
through surgical	Futura wrist brace
appliance	
departments at	
most district	
hospitals)	

Head supports   Soft felt collar
SALT head support
  available privately from:
    Salts
    Saltair House
    Lord Street
    Birmingham B7 4DS
    Tel: 0121 359 5123
Headmaster collar
  available privately from:
    Clinical Engineering Designs Ltd
    Ability House
    242 Gosport Road
    Hampshire PO16 0SS
Lees head support (will need to be obtained through an orthotist)

Mobile arm supports	(available through local authority wheelchair service, following assessment, or can be purchased privately from QED)
Powered mobile arm supports	(available privately from Brunel University, Uxbridge, London)
Electric page turner	(available from QED)
Hoists	Oxford Mini 125 (for use within the home)
	Ceiling track – contact local occupational therapist for information
Slings	Quick-fit hammock with head support

Major adaptations

For details of expensive major equipment, stair lifts, through-floor lifts, ramps, bathroom alterations, building extensions it is advisable to contact the local community occupational therapist before considering purchase.

Driving

Motability   (see Appendix C)
Driving assessments:
    Mobility Centre
    Banstead
    Damson Way
    Orchard Hill
    Queen Mary's Avenue
    Carshalton
    Surrey SM5 4NR
    Tel: 0181 770 1151

Seating

Armchairs	Electric riser/recliner (available from Hemco and Keep Able – addresses p.174)
Pressure-relief seating	Spenco Silcore
	Propad
	Sumed – Ultra 90 and Maxitec
	Roho
	Jay
	Ripple – Talley Group Ltd

Feeding

Adapted cutlery	Ultralite
Plate guard	
Dycem non-slip mat	
Plate warmer	
Drinking aids	Beakers with lids
	Electrically operated, e.g. autosip (details from Brunel University)
	Plastic drinking straws
	Pat Saunders non-return straw
Portable suction machine	(available from the MNDA)

Toileting

Raised toilet seat
Toilet frame
Grab rails

Integral toilet
frame and seat, e.g.
Scandia
Closomat Samoa –
wash/dry toilet
Medic-loo – wash/
dry toilet top
Mayfair commode/
glideabout chair
Chiltern commode/
shower chair

Showers	Level access, adapted
	Shower seat
	Integral shower/seat unit
Bathing	Non-slip mat
	Bath board
	Bath seat
	Grab rails
	Dipper portable mechanical bath lift
	Auto lift
	Electric bath lifts – Marina and Mangar

Teeth

Lightweight elec-
tric tooth brush

Beds

Marcon bed
elevator
Marcon unibed
(turning bed)
available from
    Turnblade Ltd
    Marcon Division
    PO Box 31
    Dorking RH5 5SU
    Tel: 01306 97382
Electrically oper-
ated multi-position
beds

Pressure-relieving	Spenco
mattresses	Propad

Ripple – Large Cell
Pegasus

Communication

Alphabet cards (available from the Chest, Heart and Stroke
Association)
CHSA House
123–127 Whitecross Street
London EC1Y 8JJ
Eye pointing frame E Tran Frame (available from QED)
Canon communi-
cator (available
from Easiaids)
Lightwriters SL4 Keyboard only
SL4a Keyboard and scan
SL8 (Scan only)
available from
QED, or direct
from
Toby Churchill Ltd.
20 Panton Street
Cambridge CB2 1HP
Tel: 01223 316117
Possum scanning aid (address below)
ORAC
Computer system and software (needs professional assessment by a centre
for human communication to ensure correct hardware and software are
purchased)

Environmental control systems

Possum – ECS and
communication
facility
Possum Controls Limited
Middlegreen Road
Langley
Slough
Berks SL3 6DF
Tel: 01753 79234

Steeper – ECS only
    Hugh Steeper Ltd
    Queen Mary's University Hospital
    Disability Centre
    Roehampton Lane
    London SW15 5PL
Electronic environ-
mental control
equipment, e.g.
door opener and
automatic
switching
    Ridley Electronics Ltd
    66A Clapworth Street
    Leyton
    London E10 7HA
    Tel: 0181 558 7112

Suppliers of equipment to aid independence

Hemco
Unit 59
Llandow Industrial Estate
Cowbridge
South Glamorgan CS7 7PB

Homecraft and Chester Care mail order catalogues
Sidings Road
Low Moor Estate
Kirkby-in-Ashfield
Notts NG17 7JZ
Tel: 01623 755585

Keep Able – mail order catalogue and store
Fleming Close
Park Farm
Wellingborough
Northants NN8 6UF
Tel: 01933 679426
Stores also in London and Brierley Hill, West Midlands

Nottingham Rehab – catalogue
Ludlow Hill Road
West Bridgford
Nottingham NG2 6HD
Tel: 01602 452345

Suppliers of pressure-relieving equipment

Gerald Simmonds Healthcare Ltd – Jay Cushions
9 March Place
Gatehouse Way
Aylesbury
Bucks HP19 3UG
Tel: 01296 436557

Medical Support Systems – Propad
23 Argyle Way
Ely Distribution Centre
Cardiff CF5 5NJ
Tel: 01222 595425

Pegasus
Airwave Ltd
Pegasus House
Kingscroft Court
Havant
Hants PO9 1LS
Tel: 01705 451444

Raymar – Roho Cushions
Unit 1
Fairview Estate
Reading Road
Henley-on-Thames
Oxon RG9 1HE
Tel: 01491 578446

Spenco Medical (UK) Ltd
Burrell Road
Haywards Heath
West Sussex RH16 1TW
Tel: 01444 415171

Sumed International (UK) Ltd
11 Beaumont Business Centre
Beaumont Close
Banbury
Oxon OX16 7TN
Tel: 01295 270499

Talley Group Ltd
Premier Way

Abbey Park Industrial Estate
Romsey
Hants SO51 9AQ
Tel: 01794 830702

Suppliers of professional equipment and electronics

Aremco – professional catalogue
Grove House
Lenham
Kent ME17 2PX
Tel: 01622 858502

Easiaids Limited
5 Woodcote Park Avenue
Purley
Surrey CR8 3NH
Tel: 0181 763 0203

Quest Enabling Designs (QED)
1 Prince Alfred Street
Gosport
Hampshire PO12 1QH
Tel: 01239 828444

Appendix C: Addresses

Motor Neurone Disease Associations
United Kingdom (England, Wales, Northern Ireland, the Isle of Man, Channel Islands)
PO Box 246
Northampton NN1 2PR
England
Tel: 01604 250505/22269

MNDA Helpline: 01345 626262

Scottish Motor Neurone Disease Association
50 Parnie Street
Glasgow G1 5LS
Scotland

A directory containing addresses and contact telephone numbers of Motor Neurone Disease Associations worldwide can be obtained from the Motor Neurone Disease Association, UK

Carers National Association
20–25 Glasshouse Yard
London EC1A 4JS

Citizens Advice Bureaux (National Association of)
Myddleton House
115–123 Pentonville Road
London N1 9LZ

The Compassionate Friends
53 North Street
Bedminster
Bristol BS3 1EN
(offers support and mutual friendship to bereaved parents)

Counselling (British Association for)
1 Regent Place
Rugby
Warwickshire CV21 2PJ
(directory of counselling agencies available)

Crossroads (Association of Crossroads Care Attendant Schemes)
10 Regent Place
Rugby
Warwickshire CV21 2PN

Cruse (National Organization for Bereaved People)
Cruse House
126 Sheen Road
Richmond TW9 1UR
(bereavement counselling, social support to all bereaved people)

Disabled Living Foundation
380–384 Harrow Road
London W9 2HU
(advice on daily living equipment)

Disabled Motorists Federation
National Mobility Centre
Unit 2a
Atcham Estate
Shrewsbury SY4 4UG

Leonard Cheshire Foundation
26–29 Maunsel Street
London SW1P 2QN
(provides residential, respite, domiciliary care and independent living for people with physical or mental disability)

Hospice Information Service
St Christopher's Hospice

Lawrie Park Road
London SE26 6DZ
(any information on hospice services nationally)

Motability
Gate House
Westgate
Harlow
Essex CM20 1HR

REMAP
J. J. Wright, National Organizer
Hazeldene
Ightham
Sevenoaks
Kent TN15 9AD
(makes or adapts aids for disabled people when not commercially available)

RADAR (Disability and Rehabilitation, Royal Association for)
12 City Forum
250 City Road
London EC1V 8AF
(national disability campaigning and information service)

SPOD (The Association to Aid Sexual and Personal Relationships of People with Disability)
286 Camden Road
London N7 0BJ

Voluntary Organizations, National Council for (NCVO)
Regents Wharf
8 All Saints Street
London N1 9RL

Reference

Disability Rights Handbook, 19th edition, April 1994–April 1995
Disability Alliance Educational and Research Association
Universal House
88–94 Wentworth Street
London E1 7SA

Index